Corticosteroids - A Paradigmatic Drug Class

Edited by Celso Pereira

Published in London, United Kingdom

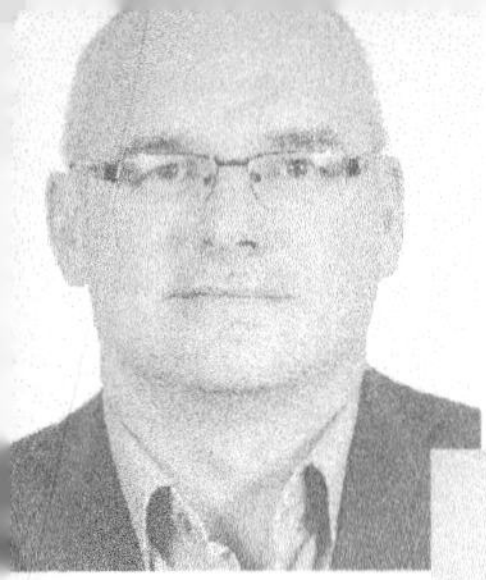

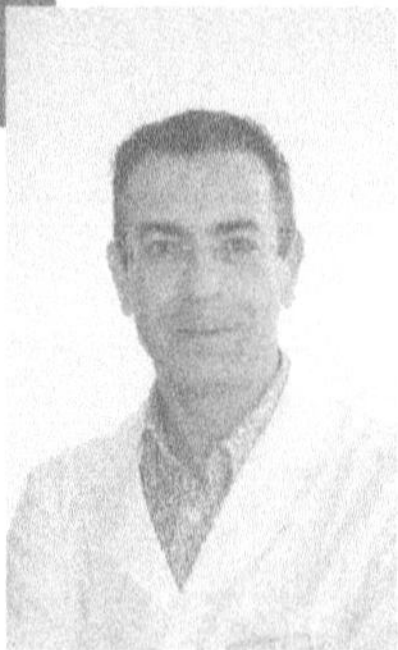

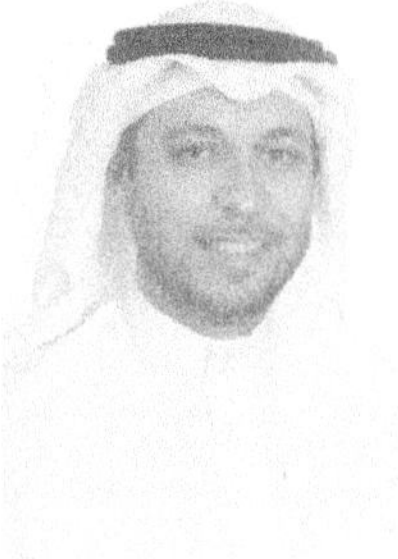

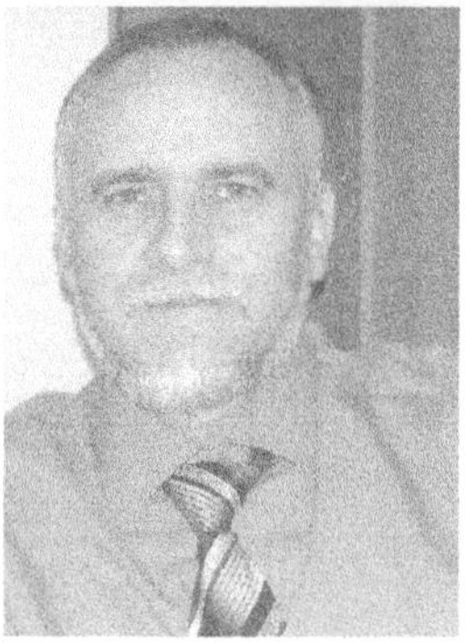

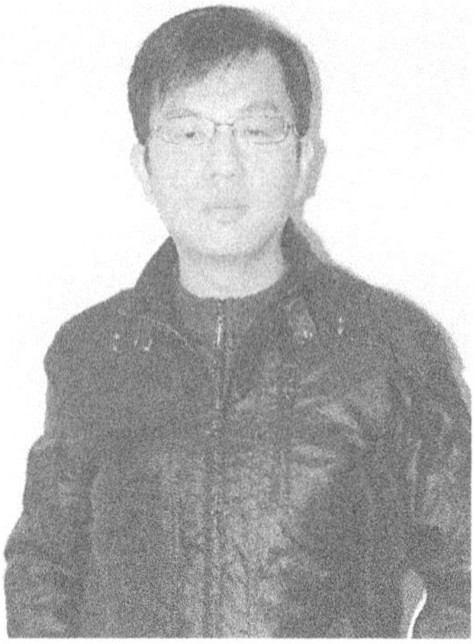

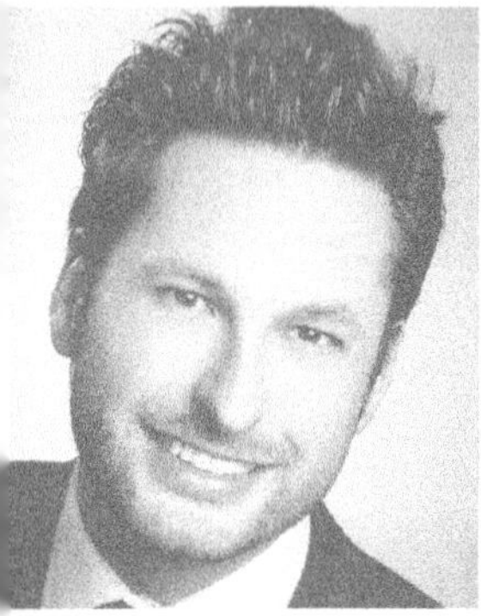

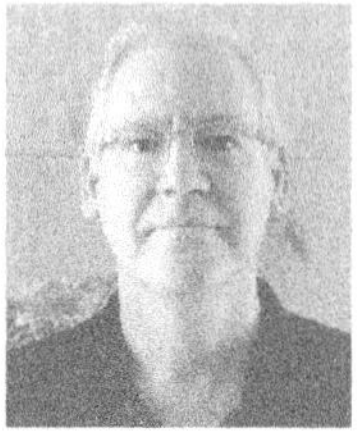

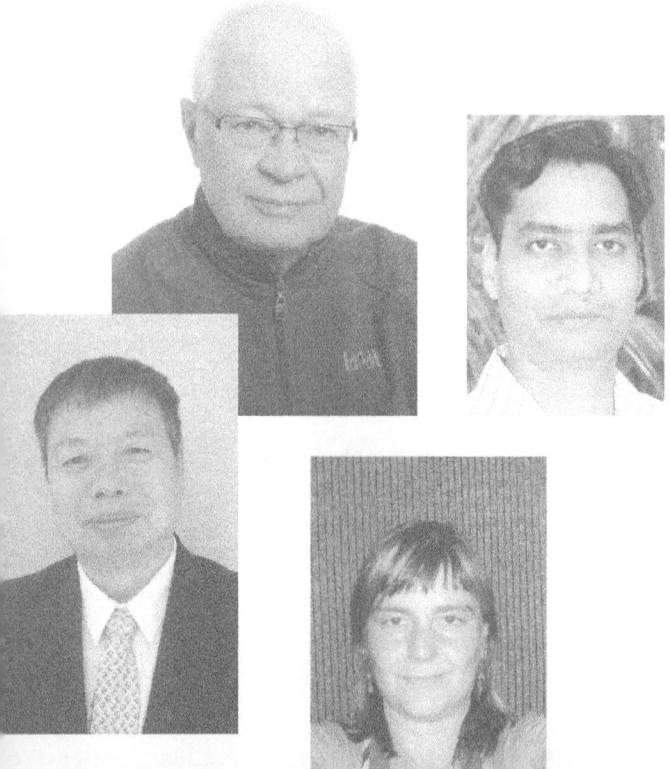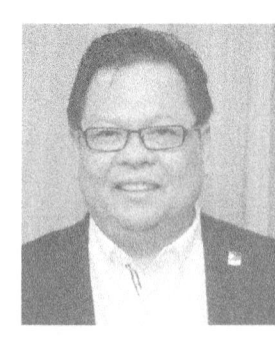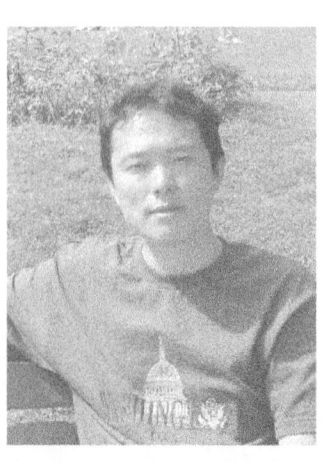

IntechOpen

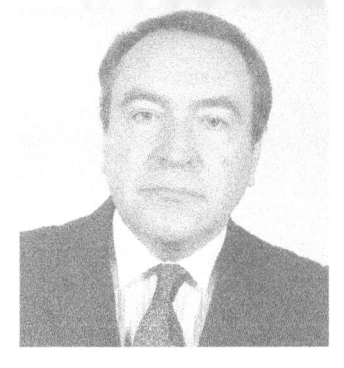
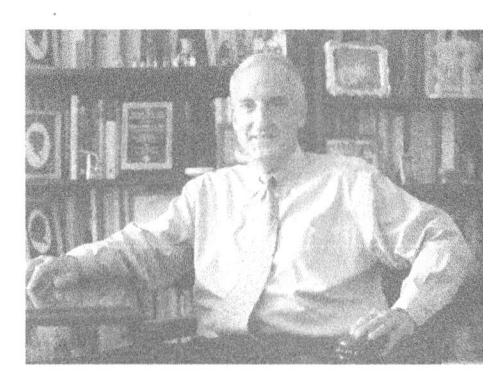
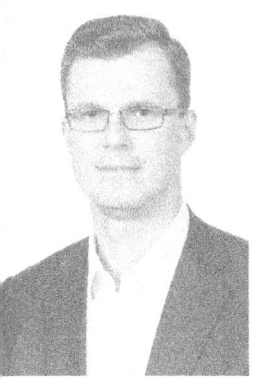
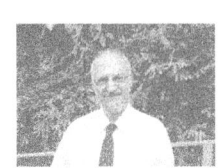
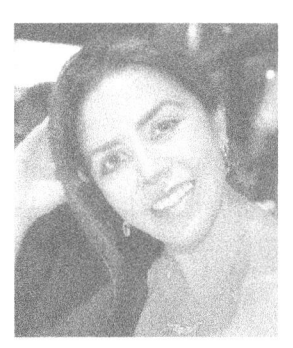

Supporting open minds since 2005

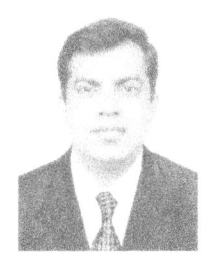
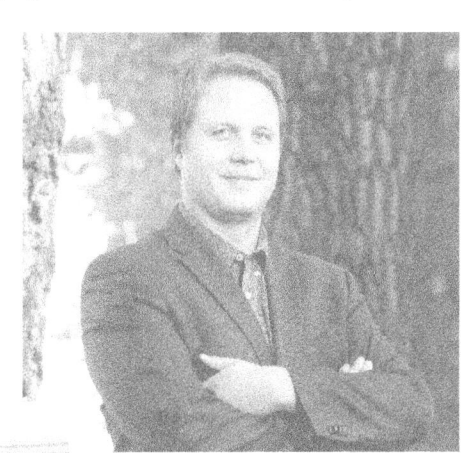
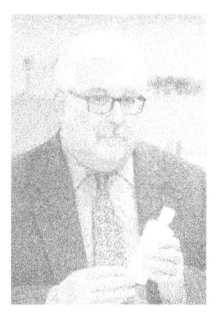
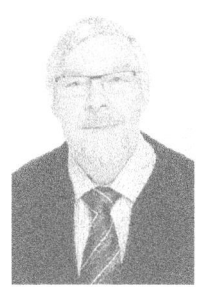
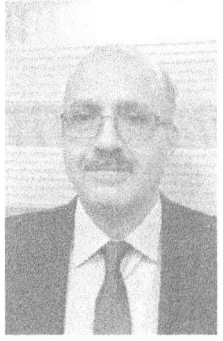
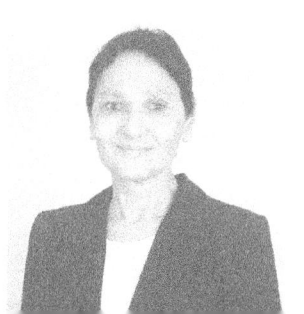
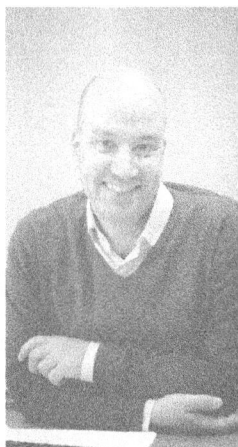

Corticosteroids - A Paradigmatic Drug Class
http://dx.doi.org/10.5772/intechopen.94686
Edited by Celso Pereira

Contributors
Michael Onyema, Magdalena B. Skarżyńska, Piotr H. Skarzynski, Alesandra Florescu, Anca Emanuela Muşetescu, Cristina Criveanu, Ana Maria Bumbea, Florin Bobîrcă, Anca Bobîrcă, Aml M. Erhuma, Sonja Pavlovic, Vladimir Gasic, Branka Zukic, Biljana Stankovic, Nikola Kotur, Djordje Pavlovic, Sunbul S. Ahmed

© The Editor(s) and the Author(s) 2021
The rights of the editor(s) and the author(s) have been asserted in accordance with the Copyright, Designs and Patents Act 1988. All rights to the book as a whole are reserved by INTECHOPEN LIMITED. The book as a whole (compilation) cannot be reproduced, distributed or used for commercial or non-commercial purposes without INTECHOPEN LIMITED's written permission. Enquiries concerning the use of the book should be directed to INTECHOPEN LIMITED rights and permissions department (permissions@intechopen.com).
Violations are liable to prosecution under the governing Copyright Law.

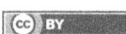

Individual chapters of this publication are distributed under the terms of the Creative Commons Attribution 3.0 Unported License which permits commercial use, distribution and reproduction of the individual chapters, provided the original author(s) and source publication are appropriately acknowledged. If so indicated, certain images may not be included under the Creative Commons license. In such cases users will need to obtain permission from the license holder to reproduce the material. More details and guidelines concerning content reuse and adaptation can be found at http://www.intechopen.com/copyright-policy.html.

Notice
Statements and opinions expressed in the chapters are these of the individual contributors and not necessarily those of the editors or publisher. No responsibility is accepted for the accuracy of information contained in the published chapters. The publisher assumes no responsibility for any damage or injury to persons or property arising out of the use of any materials, instructions, methods or ideas contained in the book.

First published in London, United Kingdom, 2021 by IntechOpen
IntechOpen is the global imprint of INTECHOPEN LIMITED, registered in England and Wales, registration number: 11086078, 5 Princes Gate Court, London, SW7 2QJ, United Kingdom
Printed in Croatia

British Library Cataloguing-in-Publication Data
A catalogue record for this book is available from the British Library

Additional hard and PDF copies can be obtained from orders@intechopen.com

Corticosteroids - A Paradigmatic Drug Class
Edited by Celso Pereira
p. cm.
Print ISBN 978-1-83969-481-3
Online ISBN 978-1-83969-482-0
eBook (PDF) ISBN 978-1-83969-483-7

We are IntechOpen,
the world's leading publisher of Open Access books
Built by scientists, for scientists

5,500+
Open access books available

136,000+
International authors and editors

170M+
Downloads

156
Countries delivered to

Our authors are among the
Top 1%
most cited scientists

12.2%
Contributors from top 500 universities

Selection of our books indexed in the Book Citation Index (BKCI)
in Web of Science Core Collection™

Interested in publishing with us?
Contact book.department@intechopen.com

Numbers displayed above are based on latest data collected.
For more information visit www.intechopen.com

Meet the editor

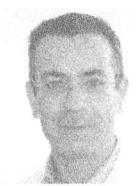

Prof. Celso Pereira, MD, Ph.D., is head-chief of the Clinical Immunology Unit and Clinical Herbal Medicine in Clinical Practice, Medicine Faculty, Coimbra University, Portugal. He is also a graduated specialist in immuno-allergy and has developed clinical activity at Coimbra Surgical Center. His main activities include clinical practice, education (pre and postgraduate), and clinical and laboratory research. He was president of the Immuno-Allergy Board of the Portuguese Medical Association. He is the coordinator of some Portuguese clinical guidelines and a member of the national committee for the diagnostic procedures for allergy and clinical immunology and the national committee for COVID vaccination. His scientific interests include research in the mechanisms of respiratory allergy, specific immunotherapy, and medicinal plant applications.

Contents

Preface XI

Chapter 1 1
The Interaction between Maternal and Fetal
Hypothalamic – Pituitary – Adrenal Axes
by Aml M. Erhuma

Chapter 2 19
Applications of Corticosteroid Therapy in Inflammatory Rheumatic
Diseases
*by Anca Emanuela Mușetescu, Cristina Criveanu, Anca Bobircă,
Alesandra Florescu, Ana-Maria Bumbea and Florin Bobircă*

Chapter 3 47
Corticosteroids in Otorhinolaryngology
by Magdalena B. Skarzynska and Piotr H. Skarzynski

Chapter 4 65
Pharmacogenomics and Pharmacotranscriptomics of Glucocorticoids
in Pediatric Acute Lymphoblastic Leukemia
*by Vladimir Gasic, Djordje Pavlovic, Biljana Stankovic, Nikola Kotur,
Branka Zukic and Sonja Pavlovic*

Chapter 5 83
Corticosteroids in Neuro-Oncology: Management of Intracranial
Tumors and Peritumoral Edema
by Sunbul S. Ahmed

Chapter 6 103
Corticosteroid Replacement Therapy
by Michael C. Onyema

Preface

Corticosteroids came into use in the late 1940s, and today they represent an irreplaceable pharmacological group for treating numerous chronic conditions.

Continued scientific research has enabled the identification of numerous broad-spectrum pharmacological mechanism signals through genomic and non-genomic pathways. The therapeutic efficacy of corticosteroids was well established in different inflammatory disorders long before many of these mechanisms were identified.

This book examines the biological intervention of endogenous steroids and their rational application for some clinical therapeutic approaches in different pathologies.

The therapeutic use of corticosteroids is not limited to the clinical applications developed in this book. Indeed, anti-inflammatory and immunosuppressive effects are crucial for a variety of disorders with expression in almost all organs and systems, namely, autoinflammatory, autoimmune, and allergic conditions, among others. This results in the availability of topical or systemic formulations, with specific and individual bioavailability, mechanisms, and adverse effects.

In current precision medicine, the re-inventive capacity of corticosteroids is remarkable, with a plethora of mechanisms and new potentials that make them a pharmacological class with unique characteristics and persistently necessary for the effective therapeutic control of more and more clinical disorders.

I would like to thank all the contributing authors for providing up-to-date reviews and new clues for future research.

Celso Pereira, MD, PhD
Clinical Immunology,
Medicine Faculty,
University of Coimbra,
Coimbra, Portugal

Chapter 1

The Interaction between Maternal and Fetal Hypothalamic – Pituitary – Adrenal Axes

Aml M. Erhuma

Abstract

The Hypothalamic – Pituitary – Adrenal (HPA) Axis is a unique system that mediates an immediate reactivity to a wide range of stimuli. It has a crucial role in synchronizing the behavioral and hormonal responses to internal and external threats, therefore, increases the chance of survival. It also enables the body systems to adapt to challenges put up by the pregnancy. Since the early stages of pregnancy and throughout delivery, HPA axis of the mother continuously navigates that of the fetus, and both have a specific cross talk even beyond the point of delivery and during postnatal period. Any disturbance in the interaction between the maternal and fetal HPA axes can adversely affect both. The HPA axis is argued to be the mechanism through which maternal stress and other suboptimal conditions during prenatal period can program the fetus for chronic disease in later life. In this chapter, the physiological and non-physiological communications between maternal and fetal HPA axes will be addressed while highlighting specific and unique aspects of this pathway.

Keywords: Hypothalamic–Pituitary–Adrenal Axis, glucocorticoids, maternal stress, fetal programming, intrauterine environment

1. Introduction

It is fundamental to know that HPA axis is considered among the few body systems that start functioning as early as 8–12 weeks of gestation [1]. This indicates that HPA axis is a vital system for fetal development, where Corticotrophin releasing hormone (CRH) and Adrenocorticotropic hormone (ACTH) are crucial for pituitary growth, adrenal cortical differentiation and maturation, as well as steroidogenesis in the fetus, which is driven mainly via Vascular Endothelial Growth Factor (VEGF) and epidermal growth factor (EGF) [2, 3]. Moreover, fetal HPA axis promotes other fetal organ structural and functional maturation such as lung, liver, gastrointestinal tract, central nervous system (CNS) and other organs important for postnatal thrive [4]. However, it has been found that early fetal environment can have detrimental effects on the proper physiological response of HPA axis, and subsequently can increase fetal risk of diseases later in life. In this chapter, possible intrauterine influences on this crucial pathway will be explored.

2. Development and Anatomy of the pituitary gland

The hypophysis is a blend of two tissues. Around week 3 of gestation, a finger of ectoderm grows upward from the roof of the mouth forming a protrusion which known as Rathke's pouch [5]. Later, this will develop into the anterior pituitary or adenohypophysis (**Figure 1A**). Simultaneously, another projection of ectodermal tissue evaginates ventrally from the diencephalon of the developing brain and form the posterior pituitary or neurohypophysis. As the fetus grows and develops, the two tissues grow into one another and become tightly apposed, but their structure remains distinctly different, reflecting their differing embryological origins (**Figure 1B**).

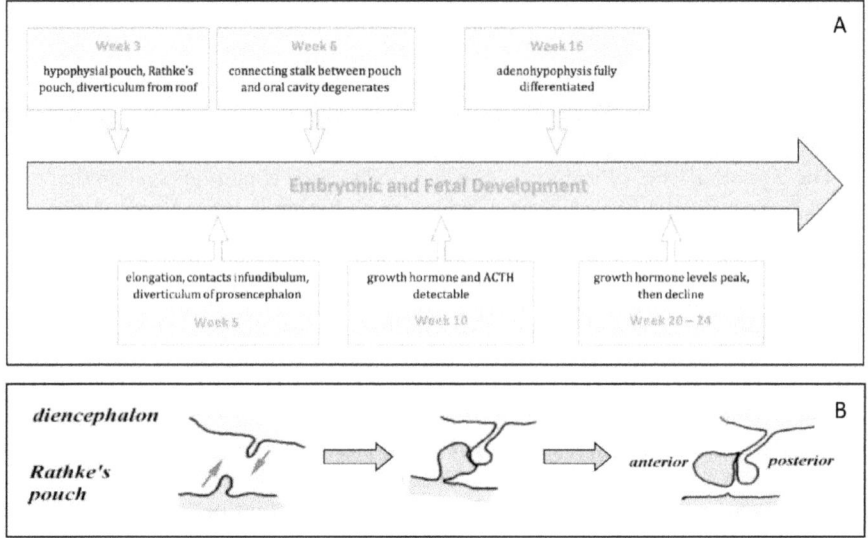

Figure 1.
(A) Timeline of fetal pituitary gland development. (B) Pituitary gland embryogenesis.

Based on the histological features, the adenohypophysis and neurohypophysis are subdivided as follow: (**Figure 2**)

- Adenohypophysis (Anterior pituitary):

  Pars distalis: It is the distal thick round part of the adenohypophysis.
  Pars tuberalis: It is the longitudinal part that surrounds the infundibular stalk.
  Pars intermedia: It is a thin layer of tissue that is separated from the pars distalis by a hypophyseal cleft.

- Neurohypophysis (Posterior pituitary):

  Pars nervosa: It is the thick, round distal part of the posterior pituitary.
  Median eminence: It is the upper section of the neurohypophysis above the pars tuberalis.

  Infundibular stalk: It is the "stem" that connects the pars nervosa to the base of the brain [6].

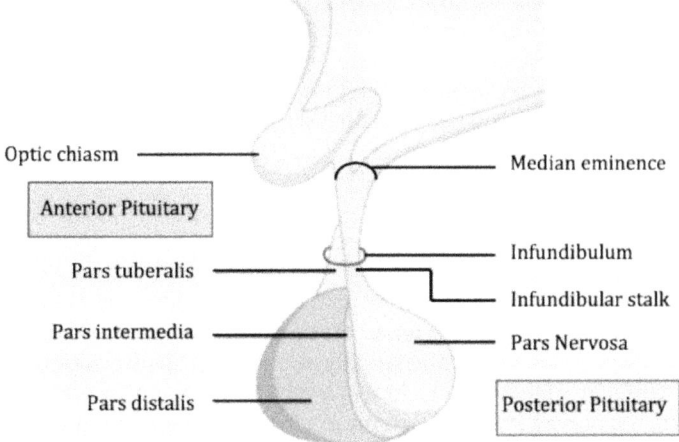

Figure 2.
Anatomy of human pituitary gland.

3. Basic regulation of HPA Axis

The HPA axis is regulated precisely and continuously. The main CNS regulation of HPA axis is through activation of corticotrophin releasing hormone (CRH) from the paraventricular nuclei (PVN) whose cell bodies are located in the hypothalamus

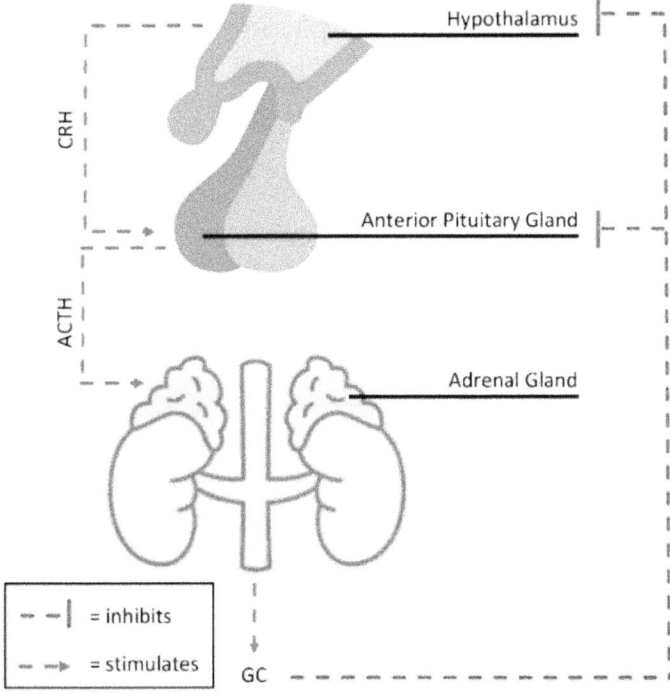

Figure 3.
Basic physiology of HPA axis regulation. CRH, corticotrophin releasing hormone; ACTH, adrenocorticotropic hormone; GC, glucocorticoids.

and also produce arginine vasopressin (AVP). Through pituitary-portal circulation in median eminence of the hypothalamus, CRH will be secreted and carried to the anterior loop of the pituitary gland. Subsequently, this will stimulate the secretion of Adrenocorticotropic hormone (ACTH) into the peripheral circulation. As a result, the adrenal cortex will be stimulated for synthesis and secretion of glucocorticoids into the blood stream (**Figure 3**) [7].

4. Circadian rhythm of cortisone secretion

The cortisone secretion in our circulation exhibits a specific regular rhythm known as the circadian rhythm (**Figure 4**). This is because plasma cortisone level will be high in early morning and gradually decreases in the circulation as we approach the night, and reaches its lowest level, the nadir, during early hours of our sleep. Then, the plasma level of cortisone gradually increases to return to its high level. This pattern can be disrupted by many factors such as stress, disease, exercise, and during physiological adaptation to pregnancy.

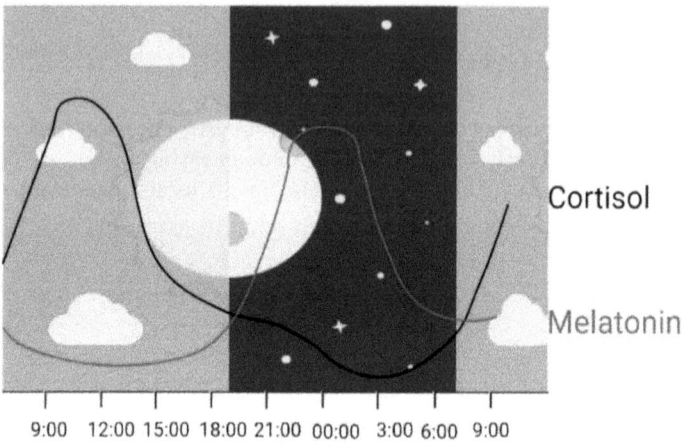

Figure 4.
Circadian rhythm of cortisol secretion.

5. Molecular mechanism of glucocorticoid action

The glucocorticoid receptor (GR), a member of the nuclear steroid receptor superfamily that acts as a ligand-dependent transcription factor to regulate the expression of glucocorticoid-responsive genes [8].

The GR can activate or suppress gene expression depending on the glucocorticoid response element sequence in the promoter region of GR responsive genes or binding DNA indirectly via other transcription factors (**Figure 5**). The association of GR with various cell types, such as ovary, suggests that it has a direct impact on gonadal reproduction [9, 10].

Glucocorticoid receptors are usually found in the cytoplasm as a complex with heat shock proteins (HSP) 90, 70, and 23. When the glucocorticoids are secreted from the adrenal cortex, they enter the target cell cytoplasm and mobilize the HSP to bind the GR. This complex will then be translocated to the nucleus,

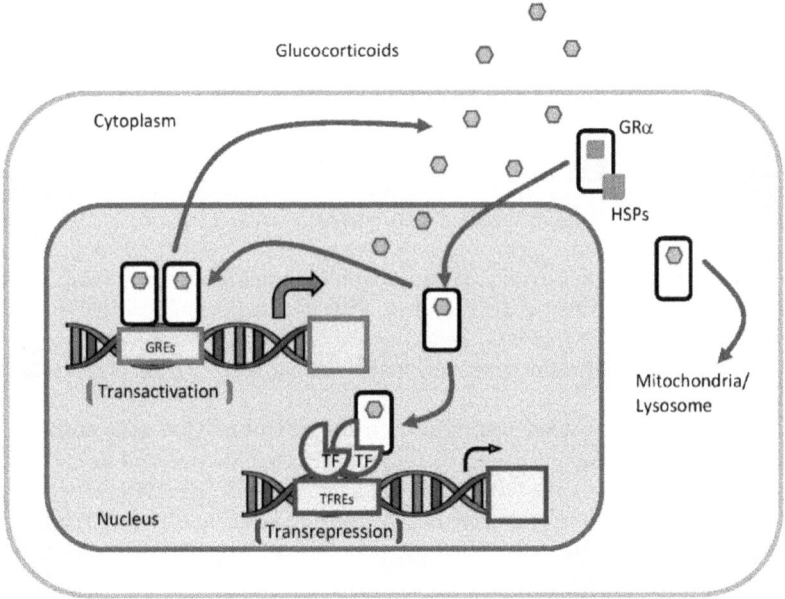

Figure 5.
Molecular mechanism of glucocorticoid action. GRα, glucocorticoid receptor alpha; HSPs, heat shock proteins; GREs, glucocorticoid responsive elements; TF, transcription factor; TFREs, transcription factor responsive elements.

where it binds to a specific DNA sequence in the promotor region of the GR responsive genes, resulting in activation of gene expression via attracting other transcription factors, which will bind to the promotor region as well as RNA polymerase II. GR can also modulate target gene expression through protein–protein interaction rather than direct DNA binding [11–13].

6. Hypothalamic pituitary adrenal Axis interaction with different body systems

The HPA axis is a very complex system that plays a crucial role in many physiological and pathological processes in the human body. One of earliest evidence that has led to the discovery of adrenal hormones and its fundamental functions was dated back to 1855 [14]. Thomas Addison found that adrenal insufficiency was associated with a group of manifestations that indicate dysfunction of other systems. Among these manifestations is excess of circulating lymphocytes. This has been confirmed in other studies that show adrenal gland removal will eventually result in thymus gland hypertrophy [15]. Hence, the wide pharmacological use of glucocorticoids to suppress the immune response in severe inflammation and anaphylactic reaction is mainly based on this interaction between the immune system and the HPA axis. Moreover, Addison noted that other systems involved include the gastrointestinal system (nausea, vomiting, loss of appetite and abdominal pain), cardiovascular system (hypotension), musculoskeletal system (muscle and joint pain and extreme fatigue), integumentary system (hyperpigmentation and hair loss), nervous system (irritability, depression and behavioral abnormality) and endocrine system (hypoglycemia).

7. Interaction between HPA Axis and reproductive hormones

It has been found that the HPA axis exhibits inhibitory effects on the female reproductive system through the inhibitory effects of CRH and CRH-induced proopiomelanocortin peptides on the hypothalamic gonadotropin-releasing hormone secretion. Moreover, glucocorticoids will suppress pituitary secretion of luteinizing hormone (LH) as well as ovarian production of estradiol and progesterone, with increased peripheral tissue estrogen resistance. Therefore, it was evident that stress, eating disorders, chronic excessive exercise, melancholic depression, chronic alcoholism, and Cushing disease result in patients suffering from amenorrhea, known as hypothalamic amenorrhea. This is characterized by low follicular stimulating hormone (FSH), LH, Estradiol (E2) and progesterone, associated with anovulation at the same time, and hence the name hypo-gonadotrophic hypogonadism.

On the other hand, estrogen is a profound stimulator of CRH gene promotor region and will, therefore, cause an increase in CRH production and its end-product, cortisone, rendering the female body in a hypercortisolism state, especially around the ovulation time of the menstrual cycle and during the early stages of pregnancy.

Reproductive tissue is found to be under the influence of the local HPA axis hormones. The ovaries and the endometrium both contain CRH and its receptors as autocoid regulators. These HPA axis components are crucial in the ovulatory process, corpus luteum lysis, endometrial shedding in menstruation, and blastocyst endometrial implantation, if pregnancy occurs. Placental CRH plays an important role in the adaptation of other systems to pregnancy and acts as a parturition clock, involved in the initiation of labor [16].

The Gonadal function is under the influence of the hypothalamic–pituitary-gonadal (HPG) axis, which is run just parallel to HPA axis. In the HPG axis, the Gonadotrophin-releasing hormone (GnRH) released from the hypothalamus will be transported by the portal circulation to the anterior pituitary to enhance and cause the release of gonadotrophic hormone, FSH, and LH. FSH will bind its receptors and promote granulosa cell growth and release of estradiol and other hormones like inhibin, activin and follistatin. Whereas LH will promote the oocyte maturation, ovulation, and corpus luteum luteinization. High levels of circulating estrogen and progesterone can cause negative feedback inhibition on hypothalamic release of GnRH and pituitary production of FSH and LH. In situations of high glucocorticoid release, as in stress or in Cushing disease, the individual will suffer from hypogonadotropic hypogonadism. Glucocorticoids cause gonadal dysfunction through binding to glucocorticoid receptors in the hippocampus region of the brain and will, subsequently, affect the individual behavior and cause inhibition of GnRH release. This will lead to a significant reduction in FSH and LH production with subsequent decrease in circulating estrogen and progesterone hormones. Glucocorticoids impact the ovaries directly by inhibiting steroid hormone synthesis or causing glucocorticoid-induced apoptosis [17, 18].

8. HPA Axis during pregnancy and labor

It is clear now that HPA axis interacts with the reproductive hormones and plays an essential role in the normal menstrual cycle, ovulation, and embryo endometrial implantation. However, this interplay is very precise, necessitating a balance between the levels of the glucocorticoids and reproductive hormones to maintain normal fertility and reproductivity of the human being.

During early pregnancy, in human, the cortisol level is lower than that in late pregnancy. As the pregnancy continues, the cortisol level increases, resulting in a greater difference between nadir and peak. The lower levels of glucocorticoids in early pregnancy are suggested to facilitate the blastocyst implantation in the endometrium, as evidenced by higher salivary cortisol levels 1–3 weeks post-conception found in women with miscarriage when compared to those with continuous pregnancy.

Women with chronic stress in early pregnancy have been noted to have blunting of cortisol levels in the morning, with no change in the nadir point of the circadian rhythm. As pregnancy progresses to mid and late gestation, HPA control will be altered and hypo-responsiveness to stress will also be evident. Unfortunately, the placental production of HPA peptides will challenge precise maternal HPA axis function assessment [19, 20].

However, in animal studies, in early pregnancy, the basal and stress-exposed HPA axis activities were found to be similar to non-pregnant animals. Nonetheless, in late pregnancy, pregnant rats show reduced basal activity of HPA axis in addition to less reactivity to stress exposure. The hypo-responsiveness in late pregnancy has been investigated in animal models. In rats, the decreased HPA axis activity and hypo-responsiveness to stress in late pregnancy could be due to attenuated vasopressin secretion from the hypothalamus with maintained CRH. The lack of augmenting vasopressin effect will result in a weak response of the anterior pituitary to CRH and subsequently, less ACTH release in basal conditions and upon stress exposure. Moreover, there will be reduced excitatory input signals from the stress processing network in the limbic forebrain, brainstem and other brain centers delivered to PVN in the hypothalamus. On the other hand, some other experimental studies on rats found that progesterone neuropeptide metabolite, allopregnanolone, exhibits an inhibitory effect on HPA axis. Allopregnanolone level is higher in late pregnancy than in early pregnancy due to higher levels of circulating progesterone hormone [21]. Other research groups have postulated that an increased level of circulating cortisol in maternal circulation towards the end of the pregnancy downregulates the hypothalamic CRH release and mediates hypo-responsiveness to stress [22–24]. This HPA axis hypo-responsiveness to stress during late pregnancy could be a biological defense mechanism to maintain the fetus in a safe environment, clear of any detrimental effect of stress-induced high glucocorticoid secretion [21, 25].

The fetus, also, protected from the unwanted effects of high maternal glucocorticoids by placental 11 β Hydroxysteroid dehydrogenase B2 enzyme (11β HSDB2) (**Figure 6**). This enzyme is responsible for inactivating 80–90% of maternal cortisol to inactive cortisone before delivering it to the fetal circulation. Despite all these natural mechanisms to minimize fetal overexposure to maternal glucocorticoids, these mechanisms fail to offer such protection during maternal stress, infection, and inflammation. Maternal and amniotic fluid (fetal) cortisol levels were both found to have a positive correlation, indicating that any increase in maternal serum cortisol level will be associated with some degree of fetal cortisol levels as well (as measured by amniotic fluid) [26].

Interestingly, it has been found across different species, including human, that ACTH and cortisol are increased on the day of parturition [27–35]. During the first and second stages of labor (cervical dilation and fetal expulsion, respectively), there will be high maternal HPA axis hormones [28, 36–39]. This could be contributed to by increased endometrial and placental CRH and ACTH, which subsequently induces fetal HPA axis hormones secretion, including ACTH and cortisol, during the third trimester of pregnancy and up to the time of delivery. The unique biological role of placental CRH is to act as a stopwatch for pregnancy and determine the labor initiation

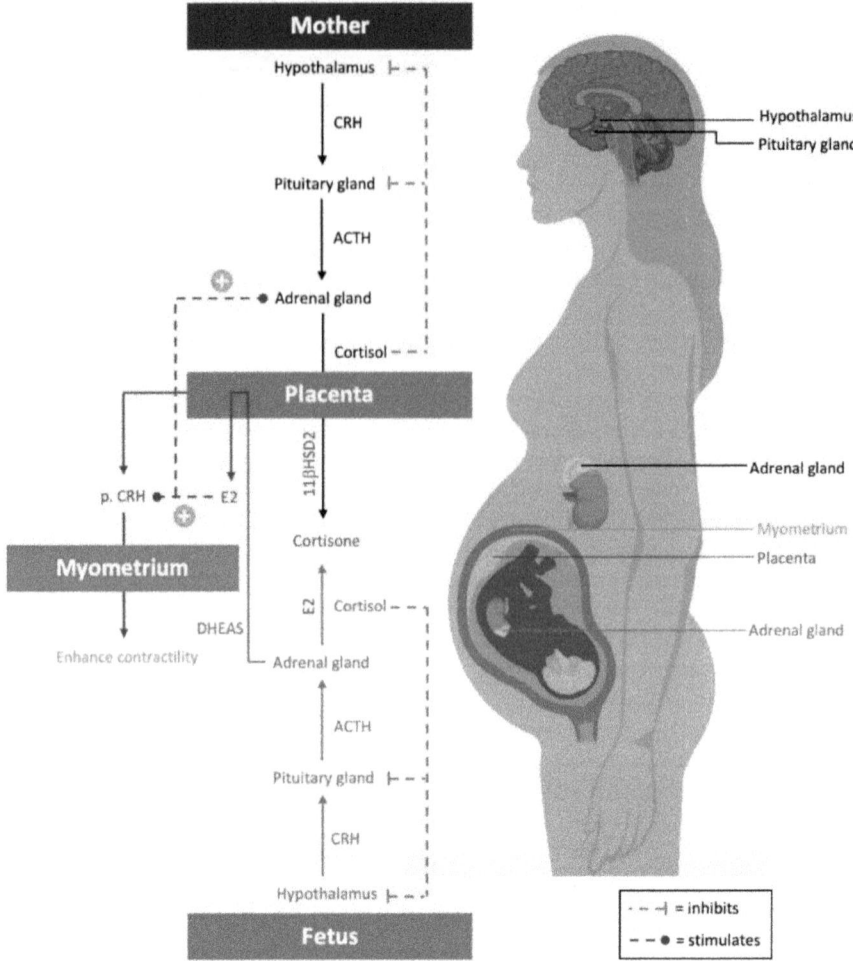

Figure 6.
Interaction of maternal and fetal HPA axes during pregnancy.

timing [40–42]. This was suggested by many studies which found an exponential increase of placental CRH in maternal and fetal circulation as pregnancy progresses (**Figure 7**). Moreover, higher levels of placental CRH in maternal circulation are associated with preterm delivery, whereas pregnant women with lower levels have longer pregnancy.

The placental CRH is a weak stimulator of maternal pituitary ACTH, therefore, the exponential increase in placental CRH levels is not associated with an equivalent increase in maternal cortisol levels. However, the main effect of placental CRH would be exerted on the myometrial responsiveness to the uterotonic effect of oxytocin and prostaglandin F2α (PGF2α). This effect of CRH is suggested to be through the reduction in C-AMP in the myometrium. It also acts as a potent vasodilator of feto-placental vessels, adding more efficacy in delivering oxytocin and prostaglandin to the myometrium and enhancing the contractility [1]. Whereas in fetal circulation, it acts directly on the fetal pituitary gland, stimulating ACTH release with subsequent increase in cortisol and dehydroepiandrosterone sulphate (DHEAS) release from fetal adrenal glands. This increase in fetal cortisol level is

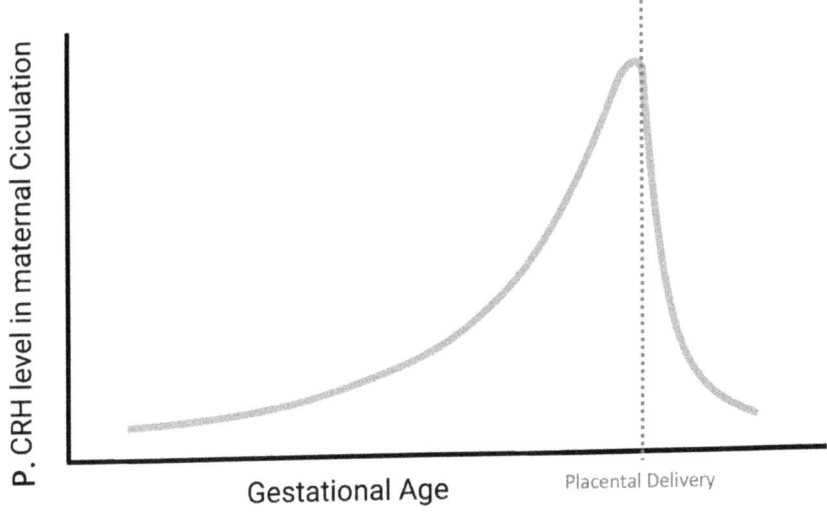

Figure 7.
Placental CRH exponential increase in maternal circulation as pregnancy progress.

essential for fetal lung maturity and alveolar surfactant production. It also induces more placental CRH production that initiate parturition onset [3, 43].

9. HPA Axis during lactation

After placental delivery, the placental-CRH levels fall sharply in the maternal circulation leading to a reduction in maternal cortisol levels (**Figure 7**). However, because there will be no change in glucocorticoid binding protein (GBP), the biologically active glucocorticoid level in maternal circulation will be maintained. Despite that, HPA axis will continue to be hyporesponsive to stress up to 1–3 months postpartum then gradually returns to normal function [44, 45]. In contrast, the salivary cortisol level in lactating mothers was found to be still high at 2 months after delivery [23].

Despite higher basal levels of HPA axis hormones during lactation, those women also exhibit less HPA axis responsiveness to stress. Interestingly, this blunted response to stress during lactation is more evident in multiparous rather than primiparous breast-feeding mothers [46].

The effect of lactation on modulating the HPA axis in basal status and in response to stress are postulated to be mediated through multiple neurohormonal mechanisms, one of which is low estradiol and other sex steroids. This results in loss of the induction effects of estradiol on the maternal adrenal cortex. Hence, this can be translated into lower cortisol levels in response to stress during lactation as compared to that during pregnancy [47, 48].

Moreover, suckling also can modulate HPA axis function depending on the environmental factors of the mother. Suckling can stimulate HPA axis only in the presence of the offspring and during early, but not late, lactation. This could be due to high circulating levels of oxytocin [49–51] and prolactin hormones [52, 53] during lactation. Because these hormones are known suppressors of HPA axis, they can cause a reduction in ACTH release.

Interestingly, maternal caring of the offspring during early postpartum period was associated with enhanced negative feedback inhibition of fetal hypothalamic CRH and reduced stress response behaviors [54, 55].

10. HPA Axis role in Fetal programming of adult disease

Optimal intrauterine fetal environment is pivotal for healthy fetal organ growth and maturation, hence subsequent proper function throughout the lifespan of the individual. Suboptimal conditions encountered in this environment can produce lifelong detrimental effects on the human body. This is the main concept of the fetal programming hypothesis by Barker [56, 57].

Therefore, any type of intrauterine insult can result in fetal programming of adult disease. This has been revealed by a bulk of epidemiological studies and also by many animal experimental studies. Our data from maternal low protein diet model have shown that maternal low protein diet during a specific period of gestation can program metabolic syndrome phenotype in the offspring in later life [58]. This metabolic phenotype was a result of altered expression of key lipid metabolism related genes and insulin signaling pathway. Preliminary data from our animal model and from other groups [59–61] indicates that the programming effect was through a fetal glucocorticoid overexposure secondary to placental 11 β HSD 2B downregulation [62]. In addition to its main site in the placenta, 11 β HSD 2B is also found to be expressed in a wide range of fetal tissue such as the brain and liver. Placental 11 β HSD 2B is crucial for protecting the fetus from exposure to excess maternal cortisol, however, normal expression of brain 11 β HSD 2B is found to play a fundamental role in preventing depression and other psychological disorders in later life independent from placental isoform, suggesting a tissue specific function for 11 β HSD 2B [63]. While in liver, the overexpression of 11 β HSD 1 enhances hepatic lipid deposition and other metabolic abnormalities [64]. Additionally, it has been shown that the under expression of fetal brain 11 β HSD 2B is associated with downregulation of serotonin (5-hydroxytryptamine) receptor type 1A (5 HT1A) which is, in turn, associated with psychological abnormalities in later life [63]. This can explain the association between the early separation anxiety in human infants and permanent hypercortisonemia as well as high β endorphin later in life with psychopathic manifestations [65].

With regard to metabolism, glucocorticoid excess has been linked to clinical observations associated with metabolic syndrome, such as central obesity, hypertension, hyperlipidemia, and glucose intolerance [66–68]. In liver, glucocorticoids increase the activities of enzymes involved in fatty acid synthesis and promote the secretion of lipoproteins [67, 69]. The hepatic lipogenic effect of glucocorticoids is consistent with clinical findings that glucocorticoid therapy causes triglyceride accumulation within the liver and is responsible for the non-alcoholic fatty liver disease [70, 71]. Therefore, it has been suggested that prenatal exposure to maternal glucocorticoids could be responsible, at least in part, for the development of the offspring phenotype [62].

As these adrenal hormones have powerful programming properties during the perinatal period, it can be speculated that long-term disturbances observed in offspring may be, in part, mediated by maternal glucocorticoid excess. Consistent with this hypothesis is the fact that hypertension in rats induced by maternal dietary protein restriction can be prevented by pharmacological blockade of glucocorticoid biosynthesis in the pregnant dam and her offspring, but reversed by concomitant corticosterone administration [67, 72]. In low protein animal model of adult disease, adrenalectomy resulted in the removal of the hypertensive state in a corticosterone-dependent manner [67, 73]. This animal model has shown low protein-exposed offspring developed disturbances of hypothalamic–pituitary–adrenal axis activity and up-regulation of glucocorticoid-sensitive enzymes in liver and brain [74].

Across a wide range of human epidemiological and experimental studies and other animal models of programming, the HPA axis is the universal target of the different intrauterine insults through which the programming of adult disease will be mediated [75–81].

11. Conclusion

To sum up, the HPA axis is a complex neurohormonal network that controls a vast majority of the body physiological performance. It is not surprising that the HPA axis develops very early in the embryo, at around 3 weeks of gestation and ACTH become detectable at around 10 weeks of gestation. This can be translated to the fact that the HPA axis is a crucial pathway that respond to surrounding threat to ensure survival. HPA axis has a double phase function, i.e., in-utero and ex-utero. During each phase it will interact differently with the environment. While the HPA axis is controlling the other endocrine systems in the body, however, it remains under continuous feedback loop regulation by downstream hormones. This is a precise way to maintain hormonal balance and homeostasis. During intrauterine life, the fetal HPA axis interacts with the maternal axis through the placental barrier, which is equipped with 11 β HSD enzyme, the placental security guard, allowing only 10–20% of active maternal cortisol to access the fetal circulation. Regardless of the insult encountered during intrauterine life, the HPA axis in mother and fetus will be dysregulated and the placenta barrier mechanism impaired. The detrimental effects will continue beyond the intrauterine life and will be conveyed later in adult life as cardiovascular, metabolic, and psychological diseases. Maternal stress, illness, infection, inflammation, malnutrition, and other stressors are all able to induce fetal programming of adult disease through the HPA axis. Finally, healthy lifestyle as an effective strategy in disease prevention should undoubtedly be started long before the birth of the individual. The mother should start a healthy lifestyle to ensure the wellbeing of her offspring in the adult life as soon as the pregnancy is detected.

Acknowledgements

I would like to express my appreciation to Miss Bushra M Abdallah and Miss Tasneem Othman for designing the figures used in this chapter. I would also like to thank my husband, Dr. Muftah A. Nasser, and my children, Lina, Abdulrahman, Reeman, and Mohamed for being supportive and encouraging.

Conflict of interest

The authors declare no conflict of interest.

Author details

Aml M. Erhuma
School of Biomedical Sciences, University of Nottingham, Nottingham, UK

*Address all correspondence to: aml_erhuma@yahoo.co.uk

IntechOpen

© 2021 The Author(s). Licensee IntechOpen. This chapter is distributed under the terms of the Creative Commons Attribution License (http://creativecommons.org/licenses/by/3.0), which permits unrestricted use, distribution, and reproduction in any medium, provided the original work is properly cited.

References

[1] Rose J, Schwartz J, Green J, Kerr D. Development of the corticotropin-releasing factor adrenocorticotropic hormone/beta-endorphin system in the mammalian fetus. Fetal and neonatal physiology. 1998:2431-2442.

[2] Ishimoto H, Jaffe RB. Development and function of the human fetal adrenal cortex: a key component in the feto-placental unit. Endocrine reviews. 2011;32(3):317-355.

[3] Mesiano S, Jaffe RB. Developmental and functional biology of the primate fetal adrenal cortex. Endocrine reviews. 1997;18(3):378-403.

[4] Winter JS. Fetal and neonatal adrenocortical physiology. Fetal and neonatal physiology: Elsevier; 2004. p. 1915-1925.

[5] Bancalari RE, Gregory LC, McCabe MJ, Dattani MT. Pituitary gland development: an update. Endocr Dev. 2012;23:1-15.

[6] Ilahi S, Ilahi TB. Anatomy, Adenohypophysis (Pars Anterior, Anterior Pituitary). StatPearls [Internet]. 2020.

[7] Dunn AJ. The HPA axis and the immune system: A perspective. NeuroImmune Biology. 2007;7:3-15.

[8] Nicolaides NC, Galata Z, Kino T, Chrousos GP, Charmandari E. The human glucocorticoid receptor: molecular basis of biologic function. Steroids. 2010;75(1):1-12.

[9] Schultz R, Isola J, Parvinen M, Honkaniemi J, Wikström AC, Gustafsson JA, et al. Localization of the glucocorticoid receptor in testis and accessory sexual organs of male rat. Mol Cell Endocrinol. 1993;95(1-2):115-120.

[10] Tetsuka M, Milne M, Simpson GE, Hillier SG. Expression of 11beta-hydroxysteroid dehydrogenase, glucocorticoid receptor, and mineralocorticoid receptor genes in rat ovary. Biol Reprod. 1999;60(2):330-335.

[11] Kino T. Stress, glucocorticoid hormones, and hippocampal neural progenitor cells: implications to mood disorders. Frontiers in physiology. 2015;6:230.

[12] Kino T, De Martino MU, Charmandari E, Mirani M, Chrousos GP. Tissue glucocorticoid resistance/hypersensitivity syndromes. The Journal of steroid biochemistry and molecular biology. 2003;85(2-5):457-467.

[13] Nicolaides NC, Chrousos G, Kino T. Glucocorticoid Receptor. Endotext [Internet]: MDText. com, Inc.; 2020.

[14] Addison T. On the constitutional and local effects of disease of the supura-renal capsules. Highley, London. 1855.

[15] Jaffe HL. THE INFLUENCE OF THE SUPRARENAL GLAND ON THE THYMUS: III. Stimulation of the Growth of the Thymus Gland Following Double Suprarenalectomy in Young Rats. The Journal of experimental medicine. 1924;40(6):753-759.

[16] Chrousos GP, Torpy DJ, Gold PW. Interactions between the hypothalamic-pituitary-adrenal axis and the female reproductive system: clinical implications. Annals of internal medicine. 1998;129(3):229-240.

[17] Bambino TH, Hsueh AJ. Direct inhibitory effect of glucocorticoids upon testicular luteinizing hormone receptor and steroidogenesis in vivo and in vitro. Endocrinology. 1981;108(6):2142-2148.

[18] Hsueh AJ, Erickson GF. Glucocorticoid inhibition of

FSH-induced estrogen production in cultured rat granulosa cells. Steroids. 1978;32(5):639-648.

[19] Sasaki A, TEMPST P, LIOTTA AS, MARGIORIS AN, HOOD LE, KENT SB, et al. Isolation and characterization of a corticotropin-releasing hormone-like peptide from human placenta. The Journal of Clinical Endocrinology & Metabolism. 1988;67(4):768-773.

[20] CHEN C-LC, CHANG C-C, KRIEGER DT, BARDIN CW. Expression and regulation of proopiomelanocortin-like gene in the ovary and placenta: comparison with the testis. Endocrinology. 1986;118(6):2382-2389.

[21] Concas A, Mostallino M, Porcu P, Follesa P, Barbaccia M, Trabucchi M, et al. Role of brain allopregnanolone in the plasticity of γ-aminobutyric acid type A receptor in rat brain during pregnancy and after delivery. Proceedings of the National Academy of Sciences. 1998;95(22):13284-13289.

[22] De Weerth C, Buitelaar JK. Physiological stress reactivity in human pregnancy—a review. Neuroscience & Biobehavioral Reviews. 2005;29(2):295-312.

[23] Kammerer M, Adams D, Von Castelberg B, Glover V. Pregnant women become insensitive to cold stress. BMC pregnancy and childbirth. 2002;2(1):1-5.

[24] Wadhwa PD, Sandman CA, CHICZ-DeMET A, Porto M. Placental CRH modulates maternal pituitary-adrenal function in human pregnancy a. Annals of the New York Academy of Sciences. 1997;814(1):276-81.

[25] Brunton P, Russell J, Douglas A. Adaptive responses of the maternal hypothalamic-pituitary-adrenal axis during pregnancy and lactation. Journal of neuroendocrinology. 2008;20(6):764-776.

[26] Duthie L, Reynolds RM. Changes in the maternal hypothalamic-pituitary-adrenal axis in pregnancy and postpartum: influences on maternal and fetal outcomes. Neuroendocrinology. 2013;98(2):106-115.

[27] Neumann I, Johnstone H, Hatzinger M, Liebsch G, Shipston M, Russell J, et al. Attenuated neuroendocrine responses to emotional and physical stressors in pregnant rats involve adenohypophysial changes. The Journal of physiology. 1998;508(1):289-300.

[28] Carr BR, Parker Jr CR, Madden JD, MacDonald PC, Porter JC. Maternal plasma adrenocorticotropin and cortisol relationships throughout human pregnancy. American journal of obstetrics and gynecology. 1981;139(4):416-422.

[29] Douglas AJ, Brunton PJ, Bosch OJ, Russell JA, Neumann ID. Neuroendocrine responses to stress in mice: hyporesponsiveness in pregnancy and parturition. Endocrinology. 2003;144(12):5268-5276.

[30] Boulfekhar L, Brudieux R. Peripheral concentrations of progesterone, cortisol, aldosterone, sodium and potassium in the plasma of the Tadmit ewe during pregnancy and parturition. Journal of Endocrinology. 1980;84(1):25-33.

[31] Brooks A, Challis J. Regulation of the hypothalamic–pituitary–adrenal axis in birth. Canadian journal of physiology and pharmacology. 1988;66(8):1106-1112.

[32] Lye S, Freitag C. Local and systemic control of myometrial contractile activity during labour in the sheep. Reproduction. 1990;90(2):483-492.

[33] Lawrence AB, Petherick J, McLean K, Deans L, Chirnside J, Gaughan A, et al. The effect of

environment on behaviour, plasma cortisol and prolactin in parturient sows. Applied Animal Behaviour Science. 1994;39(3-4):313-330.

[34] Gilbert C, Boulton M, Forsling M, Goode J, McGrath T. Restricting maternal space during parturition in the pig. Effects on oxytocin, vasopressin and cortisol secretion following vagino-cervical stimulation and administration of naloxone. Animal reproduction science. 1997;46(3-4):245-259.

[35] Jarvis S, Lawrence A, McLean K, Chirnside J, Deans L, Calvert S. The effect of environment on plasma cortisol and β-endorphin in the parturient pig and the involvement of endogenous opioids. Animal Reproduction Science. 1998;52(2):139-151.

[36] Bacigalupo G, Langner K, Schmidt S, Saling E. Plasma immunoreactive beta-endorphin, ACTH and cortisol concentrations in mothers and their neonates immediately after delivery—their relationship to the duration of labor. 1987.

[37] Fajardo M, Florido J, Villaverde C, Oltras C, Gonzalez-Ramirez A, Gonzalez-Gomez F. Plasma levels of β-endorphin and ACTH during labor and immediate puerperium. European Journal of Obstetrics & Gynecology and Reproductive Biology. 1994;55(2):105-108.

[38] Chaim W, Mazor M. The relationship between hormones and human parturition. Archives of gynecology and obstetrics. 1998;262(1):43-51.

[39] Ochedalski T, Zylinska K, Laudanski T, Lachowicz A. Corticotrophin-releasing hormone and ACTH levels in maternal and fetal blood during spontaneous and oxytocin-induced labour. Eur J Endocrinol. 2001;144(2):117-121.

[40] Vitoratos N, Papatheodorou DC, Kalantaridou SN, Mastorakos G. "Reproductive" Corticotropin-Releasing Hormone. Annals of the New York Academy of Sciences. 2006;1092(1):310-318.

[41] Grammatopoulos D. Placental corticotrophin-releasing hormone and its receptors in human pregnancy and labour: still a scientific enigma. Journal of neuroendocrinology. 2008;20(4):432-438.

[42] McLean M, Bisits A, Davies J, Woods R, Lowry P, Smith R. A placental clock controlling the length of human pregnancy. Nature medicine. 1995;1(5):460-463.

[43] Smith R. Alterations in the hypothalamic pituitary adrenal axis during pregnancy and the placental clock that determines the length of parturition. Journal of reproductive immunology. 1998;39(1-2):215-220.

[44] Owens PC, Smith R, Brinsmead MW, Hall C, Rowley M, Hurt D, et al. Postnatal disappearance of the pregnancy-associated reduced sensitivity of plasma cortisol to feedback inhibition. Life Sciences. 1987;41(14):1745-1750.

[45] Magiakou M, Mastorakos G, Rabin D, Dubbert B, Gold P, Chrousos G. Hypothalamic corticotropin-releasing hormone suppression during the postpartum period: implications for the increase in psychiatric manifestations at this time. The Journal of Clinical Endocrinology & Metabolism. 1996;81(5):1912-1917.

[46] Tu MT, Lupien SJ, Walker CD. Multiparity reveals the blunting effect of breastfeeding on physiological reactivity to psychological stress. Journal of neuroendocrinology. 2006;18(7):494-503.

[47] KITAY JI, COYNE MD, NEWSOM W, NELSON R. Relation of the ovary to

adrenal corticosterone production and adrenal enzyme activity in the rat. Endocrinology. 1965;77(5):902-908.

[48] Figueiredo HF, Ulrich-Lai YM, Choi DC, Herman JP. Estrogen potentiates adrenocortical responses to stress in female rats. American Journal of Physiology-Endocrinology and Metabolism. 2007;292(4):E1173-E1E82.

[49] Chiodera P, Salvarani C, Bacchi-Modena A, Spallanzani R, Cigarini C, Alboni A, et al. Relationship between plasma profiles of oxytocin and adrenocorticotropic hormone during suckling or breast stimulation in women. Hormone Research in Paediatrics. 1991;35(3-4):119-123.

[50] Amico JA, Johnston JM, Vagnucci AH. Suckling-induced attenuation of plasma cortisol concentrations in postpartum lactating women. Endocrine research. 1994;20(1):79-87.

[51] Legros J-J. Inhibitory effect of oxytocin on corticotrope function in humans: are vasopressin and oxytocin ying–yang neurohormones? Psychoneuroendocrinology. 2001;26(7):649-655.

[52] Torner L, Toschi N, Pohlinger A, Landgraf R, Neumann ID. Anxiolytic and anti-stress effects of brain prolactin: improved efficacy of antisense targeting of the prolactin receptor by molecular modeling. Journal of Neuroscience. 2001;21(9):3207-3214.

[53] Donner N, Bredewold R, Maloumby R, Neumann ID. Chronic intracerebral prolactin attenuates neuronal stress circuitries in virgin rats. European Journal of Neuroscience. 2007;25(6):1804-1814.

[54] Emanuele N, Jurgens J, Halloran M, Tentler J, Lawrence A, Kelley M. The rat prolactin gene is expressed in brain tissue: detection of normal and alternatively spliced prolactin messenger RNA. Molecular endocrinology. 1992;6(1):35-42.

[55] Torner L, Maloumby R, Nava G, Aranda J, Clapp C, Neumann ID. In vivo release and gene upregulation of brain prolactin in response to physiological stimuli. European journal of neuroscience. 2004;19(6):1601-1608.

[56] Barker DJ, Eriksson JG, Forsén T, Osmond C. Fetal origins of adult disease: strength of effects and biological basis. International journal of epidemiology. 2002;31(6):1235-1239.

[57] Barker DJP. Mothers, babies and health in later life 2nd ed. Churchill Livingstone: Edinburgh. 1998.

[58] Erhuma A, Bellinger L, Langley-Evans SC, Bennett AJ. Prenatal exposure to undernutrition and programming of responses to high-fat feeding in the rat. British Journal of Nutrition. 2007;98(3):517-524.

[59] Langley-Evans SC. Maternal carbenoxolone treatment lowers birthweight and induces hypertension in the offspring of rats fed a protein-replete diet. Clinical Science. 1997;93(5):423-429.

[60] Bertram C, Trowern A, Copin N, Jackson A, Whorwood C. The maternal diet during pregnancy programs altered expression of the glucocorticoid receptor and type 2 11β-hydroxysteroid dehydrogenase: potential molecular mechanisms underlying the programming of hypertension in utero. Endocrinology. 2001;142(7):2841-2853.

[61] Whorwood C, Firth K, Budge H, Symonds M. Maternal undernutrition during early to midgestation programs tissue-specific alterations in the expression of the glucocorticoid receptor, 11β-hydroxysteroid dehydrogenase isoforms, and type 1 angiotensin II receptor in neonatal

sheep. Endocrinology. 2001;142(7):2854-2864.

[62] Erhuma A, McMullen S, Langley-Evans SC, Bennett AJ. Feeding pregnant rats a low-protein diet alters the hepatic expression of SREBP-1c in their offspring via a glucocorticoid-related mechanism. Endocrine. 2009;36(2):333-338.

[63] Shearer FJ, Wyrwoll CS, Holmes MC. The role of 11β-hydroxy steroid dehydrogenase type 2 in glucocorticoid programming of affective and cognitive behaviours. Neuroendocrinology. 2019;109(3): 257-265.

[64] Candia R, Riquelme A, Baudrand R, Carvajal CA, Morales M, Solís N, et al. Overexpression of 11β-hydroxysteroid dehydrogenase type 1 in visceral adipose tissue and portal hypercortisolism in non-alcoholic fatty liver disease. Liver International. 2012;32(3):392-399.

[65] Breier A. Experimental approaches to human stress research: Assessment of neurobiological mechanisms of stress in volunteers and psychiatric patients. Biological Psychiatry. 1989;26(5): 438-462.

[66] Thuzar M, Stowasser M. The mineralocorticoid receptor—an emerging player in metabolic syndrome? Journal of Human Hypertension. 2021:1-7.

[67] Erhuma A. Effects of maternal low-protein diet during pregnancy on lipid metabolism and gene expression in the offspring: University of Nottingham; 2006.

[68] Wang M. The role of glucocorticoid action in the pathophysiology of the metabolic syndrome. Nutrition & metabolism. 2005;2(1):1-14.

[69] Wang C-N, McLeod RS, Yao Z, Brindley DN. Effects of dexamethasone on the synthesis, degradation, and secretion of apolipoprotein B in cultured rat hepatocytes. Arteriosclerosis, thrombosis, and vascular biology. 1995;15(9):1481-1491.

[70] Woods CP, Hazlehurst JM, Tomlinson JW. Glucocorticoids and non-alcoholic fatty liver disease. The Journal of steroid biochemistry and molecular biology. 2015;154:94-103.

[71] D'souza AM, Beaudry JL, Szigiato AA, Trumble SJ, Snook LA, Bonen A, et al. Consumption of a high-fat diet rapidly exacerbates the development of fatty liver disease that occurs with chronically elevated glucocorticoids. American Journal of Physiology-Gastrointestinal and Liver Physiology. 2012;302(8):G850-GG63.

[72] Langley-Evans SC. Hypertension induced by foetal exposure to a maternal low-protein diet, in the rat, is prevented by pharmacological blockade of maternal glucocorticoid synthesis. Journal of hypertension. 1997;15(5): 537-544.

[73] Gardner DS, Jackson AA, Langley-Evans SC. Maintenance of maternal diet-induced hypertension in the rat is dependent on glucocorticoids. Hypertension. 1997;30(6):1525-1530.

[74] Langley-Evans SC, Gardner DS, Jackson AA. Maternal protein restriction influences the programming of the rat hypothalamic-pituitary-adrenal axis. The Journal of nutrition. 1996;126(6):1578-1585.

[75] Weinberg J, Sliwowska JH, Lan N, Hellemans K. Prenatal alcohol exposure: Foetal programming, the hypothalamic-pituitary-adrenal axis and sex differences in outcome. Journal of neuroendocrinology. 2008;20(4): 470-488.

[76] Meaney MJ, Szyf M, Seckl JR. Epigenetic mechanisms of perinatal

programming of hypothalamic-pituitary-adrenal function and health. Trends in molecular medicine. 2007;13(7):269-277.

[77] Romeo RD. Pubertal maturation and programming of hypothalamic–pituitary–adrenal reactivity. Frontiers in neuroendocrinology. 2010;31(2):232-240.

[78] Kapoor A, Petropoulos S, Matthews SG. Fetal programming of hypothalamic–pituitary–adrenal (HPA) axis function and behavior by synthetic glucocorticoids. Brain research reviews. 2008;57(2):586-595.

[79] Anacker C, O'Donnell KJ, Meaney MJ. Early life adversity and the epigenetic programming of hypothalamic-pituitary-adrenal function. Dialogues in clinical neuroscience. 2014;16(3):321.

[80] Jellyman J, Valenzuela O, Fowden A. Horse species symposium: glucocorticoid programming of hypothalamic-pituitary-adrenal axis and metabolic function: animal studies from mouse to horse. Journal of animal science. 2015;93(7):3245-3260.

[81] Xiong F, Zhang L. Role of the hypothalamic–pituitary–adrenal axis in developmental programming of health and disease. Frontiers in neuroendocrinology. 2013;34(1):27-46.

Chapter 2

Applications of Corticosteroid Therapy in Inflammatory Rheumatic Diseases

Anca Emanuela Mușetescu, Cristina Criveanu, Anca Bobircă, Alesandra Florescu, Ana-Maria Bumbea and Florin Bobircă

Abstract

Corticosteroids still remain the anchor drugs in therapy strategies for patients with inflammatory rheumatic diseases even though new drugs such as biologic or targeted synthetic molecules have emerged in the past years, being the most commonly prescribed medicines in the world due to their powerful immune-modulating properties. In this chapter, we aim to discuss the main characteristics of the glucocorticoids, their mechanism of action and effects on the immune system given the fact that they reduce the activation, proliferation, differentiation and survival of inflammatory cells such as macrophages and lymphocytes. Nevertheless, of great importance are the indications and tapering regimens, but also the adverse effects and various methods of monitoring the corticosteroid therapy.

Keywords: corticosteroids, immune system, regimens, adverse effects

1. Introduction

The adrenal glands are composed of the medulla which secretes cathecolamines (adrenaline and noradrenaline) and the adrenal cortex which produces glucocorticoids (cortisol), mineralocorticoids such as aldosterone and andogens (dehydropiandrosterone) [1].

In the 1930s, steroidal hormones were isolated from the adrenal cortex and synthesized a years later. Several of these structures have potent anti-inflammatory properties, but they can also have important side effects. Chemical analogues with improved activity and less side effects have been discovered and are being used for the treatment of numerous inflammatory and autoimmune diseases [2].

Although glucocorticoid (GC) is the preferred classification when using exogenous agents therapeutically, corticosteroids encompass both glucocorticoid and mineralocorticoid hormones, the term corticosteroid (CS) is considered synonymous to glucocorticoid. Commercially available synthetic GC formulations come in a number of chemical compositions, potencies and half-lives.

Glucocorticoids are hormones that regulate a variety of cellular functions, including growth, homeostasis, metabolism, cognition, and inflammation. GCs are one of the most commonly prescribed medicines in the world due to their powerful immune-modulating properties [3].

2. History of corticosteroid discovery and development

Thomas Addison first described the disease named after him in 1855 in London, in which postmortem examination of patients indicated adrenal gland atrophy. The following year, in Paris, Charles Edouard Brown-Se'quard demonstrated that surgical removal of the adrenals in small animals caused muscle fatigue, respiratory insufficiency, cardiac problems and death within 12 hours [4, 5].

The Mayo Clinic's Edward C. Kendall (1886–1972) and Zurich's Tadeus Reichstein (1897–1996) continued their research. Edward Calvin Kendall isolated four steroidal compounds from adrenal extracts in 1946. He labeled them A, B, E, and F. Later that year, Sarett synthesized compound E, known as cortisone nowadays. Rheumatologist Philip Hench discovered the compound's therapeutic potential in a patient with RA [6].

On April 13, 1949, the Mayo Clinic's Proceedings of Staff Meetings confirmed the first therapeutic use of cortisone. The first patient, a 29-year-old married woman in her fourth year of rheumatoid arthritis (RA), had been chosen by Philip S. Hench (1896–1965), chief of the Rheumatology Section [7, 8]. Before September 1948, when she received the first twice daily intramuscular injections of 50 mg of cortisone, the patient had been seen at the Mayo Clinic and had received multiple prescriptions on many occasions. Subjective improvement was recorded after the second injection. Although cortisone dosage was fluctuating between 50 mg and 100 mg per day, depressive and aggressive ideation became more prevalent, despite the improving of rheumatoid symptoms by 50% [9, 10].

Thus in 1950, Hench and Kendall, along with Tadeus Reichstein, were awarded the Nobel Prize for Medicine and Physiology for isolating with success several steroid hormones from the adrenals [11].

3. Mechanisms of action

The CS exercise their effect following the passive diffusion through cellular membranes, attachment to specific intracellular receptors and the formation of a complex that will be translocated intra-nuclear and will interact directly with certain specific DNA sequences or with other transcription factors [12, 13].

CS can exercise their effect by genomic or nongenomic mechanisms. It takes at least 30 minutes for the clinical effects of a GC to appear while operating by genomic mechanisms. Nongenomic mechanisms, by which GCs function within minutes, only occur when large doses are administered, such as in pulse therapy [14].

3.1 Genomic mechanisms

The majority of glucocorticoid effects are mediated by genomic pathways, such as binding to the GC receptor in the target cells' cytoplasm. Since GCs are lipophilic and their molecular mass is low, they can easily transit through the cell membrane [15, 16].

The balance of the intracellular enzyme 11-hydroxysteroid dehydrogenase (11–HSDs) possibly influences the sensitivity of specific tissues to GCs, in addition to the tissue-specific intracellular density of GC receptors. Only the isoform of the GC receptor, which is widely distributed in all target tissues, binds to GCs. The GC receptor–GC complex is activated and subsequently transported into the nucleus. As a dimer, it binds to sites in DNA which respond to GC, thus being able to control the transcription of targeted genes. This process is termed transactivation [17].

As monomers, activated GC receptor – GC complexes interact with transcriptional factors (such as activator protein (AP)-1, interferon regulatory factor (IRF)-3, and nuclear factor-κB (NF-κB)). These transcriptional factors are prevented from binding to their consensus sites in DNA. Transrepression is a process that results in the downregulation of predominantly pro-inflammatory protein synthesis [18].

The hypothesis has been proposed that side effects of GCs may be based predominantly on transactivation, whereas the anti-inflammatory effects can be attributed to transrepression.

The binding of GC to specific sites at the DNA level, can cause suppression or stimulation of gene transcription and numerous effects on the inflammatory process such as:

- attachment at the level of promoter sites of the pro-inflammatory genes and their inhibition (interleukin (IL)-1α, IL-1β);

- recruitment of transcription factors of gene promoter domains which encode the production of anti-inflammatory factors (IKBα-transcription inhibitor factor of NF-KB, IL-10, α-2 macroglobulin, IL-1R);

- suppression of the synthesis of most pro-inflammatory cytokines through the inhibition of NF-KB or AP-1, indispensable for the transcription of inflammation mediators [19].

Consequences of GC interference with the phenomenon of gene transcription consist of: stimulation of the synthesis of angiotensin conversion enzyme or endopeptidases which neutralizes bradykinin, a central vasodilator peptide involved in the onset angioedema. Another effect is the inhibition of the synthesis of pro-inflammatory factors by the phagocytic cells through stimulating lipocortin 1 synthesis and, subsequently, inhibition of phospholipase A2 which is responsible for the synthesis of arachidonic acid at the level of membrane phospholipid, prostaglandins, leukotrienes and free oxygen radicals. Nevertheless the inhibition of cyclooxygenase (COX)-2 synthesis, the inducible form of COX, responsible for production of prostaglandins (PG) at the inflammatory site is another consequence of the GC interference with gene transcription [20].

3.2 Nongenomic mechanisms

In addition to genomic effects, GCs exert their effects through nongenomic pathways, represented by the interaction with selective membrane receptors (specific nongenomic effects) or directly on the biological membranes (nonspecific nongenomic effects).

Nongenomic effects at high doses of GCs occur much faster than genomic effects—within minutes. Membrane-bound GC receptors are one mechanism. Nongenomic actions which do not include GC receptors change cell function by physicochemical interactions with biologic membranes [21].

4. Effects on the immune system

One of the main function of GCs is the inhibition of the activation, proliferation, differentiation and survival of macrophages and T lymphocytes as well as other inflammatory cells. GCs also promote apoptosis mainly of immature and activated T cells. Changes in cytokine synthesis and secretion are primarily responsible for this activity.

B lymphocytes and neutrophils, on the other hand, are less responsive to glucocorticoids, and glucocorticoid treatment can improve their survival [22].

4.1 Leukocytes and fibroblasts

The administration of GC has an effect on the circulating neutrophil granulocytes, increasing their number in the peripheral blood. This results in decreased myelopoiesis and bone marrow release. The effects also apply to the T cells, resulting in their redistribution. The redistribution of lymphocytes has no clinical implications. This effect occurs after 4 to 6 hours of a single dose of prednisone and returns to normal within 24 hours. The activity of B cells and the synthesis of immunoglobulin are unaffected. However, the susceptibility to infection is increased due to the effects of GCs on monocytes and macrophages. These effects lead to a decrease in the expression of class II major histocompatibility complex (MHC) molecules and Fc receptors. The administration of GC also affects the fibroblasts, leading to reduced proliferation and synthesis of fibronectin and prostaglandins [23].

4.2 Cytokines

One of the most important effects of GC therapy in chronic inflammatory disorders is on cytokine synthesis and action. A wide range of cytokines are inhibited by GC administration. GCs inhibit most Th1 pro-inflammatory cytokines such as interleukins (IL-1, IL-2, IL-3, IL-6, IL-17), but also tumor necrosis factor (TNF), interferon-γ and GM-CSF. These cytokines are thought to be responsible for synovial proliferation, cartilage damage and bone deterioration in people with RA [24]. GCs have controversial effects on Th2 cytokines such as IL-4, IL-10 and IL-13, either by stimulating or having no effect on their development [25].

4.3 Pro-inflammatory enzymes

Arachidonic acid metabolism is an essential part of the inflammatory cascade. An essential part of the cascade of inflammation is the development of prostaglandins and leukotrienes, the majority of which are highly pro-inflammatory. GCs also have an effect on the inhibition of the development of COX-2 and phospholipase A2, induced by cytokines. This process is located in monocytes/macrophages, fibroblasts and endothelial cells. Furthermore, in vitro and in vivo, glucocorticoids promote the inhibition of the metalloproteinases, especially collagenase and stromelysin. These metalloproteinases are considered the key effectors of cartilage degradation induced by IL-1 and TNF [26].

4.4 Adhesion molecules and permeability factors

Pharmacologic doses of GCs significantly reduce plasma exudation and leukocyte recruitment into inflammatory sites. Adhesion molecules regulate the migration of inflammatory cells into the sites of inflammation, which is essential in chronic inflammatory diseases.

GCs also exert their effect by stimulating the expression of adhesion molecules such as intercellular adhesion molecule-1 and E-selectin through the inhibition of pro-inflammatory cytokines. GC also have an effect on the inhibition of chemotactic cytokines such as IL-8 and macrophage chemoattractant proteins which attract immune cells to the inflammatory site. The production of nitric oxide is increased in the sites with active inflammation by the pro-inflammatory cytokines, leading to an increase in blood flow, exudation and likely activation of the inflammatory response. GCs effectively inhibit the inducible form of nitric oxide synthase induced by cytokines [27].

5. Pharmacology

After administration, both orally and parenterally, absorption is rapid and subsequently CS bind to 90% of plasma proteins. The binding is mainly done by specific globulin (CBG-corticosteroid binding globulin or transcortin) and in a reduced percentage by albumin. The biologically active form is the free cortisol (10%), which achieves high concentrations in most tissues. Metabolism takes place in the liver and excretion is urinary.

Medicinal products included in this class are similar in absorption rate, with differences in half-life and intensity of anti-inflammatory effect. Depending on the duration of action, GC can be classified into short-, medium- or long-term.

The route of administration can be:

- parenteral - intravenous pulse therapy in doses of 1–2 g, in the activity periods of the disease, in patients with RA, systemic lupus erythematosus (SLE) vasculitis, or intramuscular;

- oral - usually in the case of chronic GC therapy;

- intra-articular with depot preparations with local action;

- topical with variable absorption rates [28].

Systemic administration of GC therapy can be done in high doses, for a short period, in acute situations, or chronically, with periodic dose adjustment, depending on the therapeutic response and adverse effects. Discontinuation of therapy is considered either when the maximum therapeutic effect has been reached or in case of inefficiency or severe adverse effects without response to the specific therapy [29].

The main pharmacological characteristics of GCs are illustrated in **Table 1**.

	Equivalent GC dose	Relative GC activity	Protein binding	Half-life in plasma (hours)	Biologic half-life (hours)
Short-acting					
Cortisone	25	0.8	No	0.5	8–12
Cortisol	20	1	Yes	1.5–2	8–12
Intermediate-acting					
Methylprednisolone	4	5	No	>3.5	18–36
Prednisolone	5	4	Yes	2.1–3.5	18–36
Prednisone	5	4	Yes	3.4–3.8	18–36
Triamcinolone	4	5	Yes	2–5	18–36
Long-acting					
Dexamethasone	0.75	20–30	Yes	3–4.5	36–54
Betamethasone	0.6	20–30	Yes	3–5	36–54

Table 1.
Characteristics of main GCs.

6. Indications and dosing

Glucocorticoid therapy is indicated in multiple rheumatic diseases. In pathologies such as inflammatory myopathies, polymyalgia rheumatic, but also in systemic vasculitis, GCs are considered the focal point of the therapeutic strategy.

On the other hand, in systemic scleroderma, GCs are contraindicated in high doses, due to the increased risk of scleroderma renal crisis. However, they can be of use when systemic sclerosis is complicated by myositis or interstitial lung disease. Glucocorticoids are used as an adjunctive treatment or not at all in the treatment of other diseases [30].

In RA, GCs exert their effects by complementing the disease-modifying antirheumatic drugs (DMARDs). GCs are helpful in reducing pain in osteoarthritis, although they are not administered on a regular basis, with the exception of intra-articular injections if there are symptoms of synovitis in an osteoarthritic joint.

GCs are used to treat a variety of rheumatic diseases in varying dosages. Standardization of dosing regimens has been suggested based on pathophysiologic and pharmacokinetic evidence:

- low dose - ≤ 7.5 mg prednisone equivalent per day;

- medium dose - >7.5 mg and ≤ 30 mg prednisone equivalent per day;

- high dose - > 30 mg and ≤ 100 mg prednisone equivalent per day;

- very high dose - >100 mg prednisone equivalent per day;

- pulse therapy - ≥ 250 mg prednisone equivalent per day for one or a few days [31].

7. Systemic adverse effects of glucocorticoid therapy

It is not surprising that glucocorticoids may have a wide range of side effects given their diverse pathways and sites of action. The majority of these side effects are unavoidable, but the risk of most complications is dose and time dependent and lowering GC dosage reduces the risk of complications [32].

7.1 Risk of infections

In vitro, glucocorticoids reduce neutrophil phagocytosis and bacterial destruction, but natural bactericidal and phagocytic activities are found in vivo. Monocytes are however more susceptible; bactericidal and fungicidal activity in vivo and in vitro is decreased during treatment with medium to large doses of glucocorticoids. These variables can have an impact on the risk of infection. Therapy with a daily dosage of less than 10 mg of prednisolone or its equivalent seems to have little or only a mild elevated risk of infection, while treatment with doses of 20 to 40 mg daily seems to have an increased risk of infection. However, if the dosage and duration of therapy is prolonged, the risk of infection also rises [33].

7.2 Cardiovascular adverse effects

Some glucocorticoids seem to have mineralocorticoid effects, such as decreased sodium and chloride excretion and increased potassium, calcium, and phosphate excretion. Edema, weight gain, high blood pressure and heart complications are also possible side effects of this action. Reduced sodium and chloride excretion can result in heart failure.

Patients with inflammatory diseases have been linked to accelerated atherosclerosis and increased cardiovascular risk. Cardiovascular mortality is linked to the length of the disorder and the use of glucocorticoids. Because of their potentially harmful effects on lipids, glucose tolerance, insulin production and resistance, blood pressure and obesity, GCs can increase cardiovascular risk [34].

In vitro, GCs were found to suppress macrophage aggregation in damaged arterial walls, potentially reducing the local inflammatory response. Low-dose glucocorticoids can also improve inflammatory disease-related dyslipidemia. Low-dose GCs, on the other hand, are likely to have different effects on lipids and other cardiovascular risk factors in inflammatory disorders than medium and large doses of GCs.

Thus, in addition to conventional cardiovascular risk factors such as diabetes mellitus, length and level of inflammatory disease involvement, and co-therapies such as COX-2 selective NSAIDs, moderate and high glucocorticoid doses and long duration of therapy seem to be the most significant cardiovascular risk factors [35].

7.3 Osteoporosis

GC therapy directly influences osteoblasts, osteocytes and osteoclasts, reducing the process of bone formation and accelerating bone resorption.

Glucocorticoid receptors are located exclusively in osteoblasts, not in osteoclasts, the proliferation of the latter being the consequence of inhibition of osteoprotegerin synthesis (inhibitor of osteoclast differentiation in hematopoietic cells) and stimulation of RANK production, necessary for the osteoclastogenesis. High doses of GC also stimulate RANKL synthesis by osteoblast precursors, an event that activates osteoclast differentiation and the bone resorption process [36].

Other mechanisms involved are the decrease in the secretion of androgen and estrogen hormones, the increase in the serum level of parathormone (consequent to the decrease in intestinal calcium absorption and the increase in its renal elimination).

Suppression of the osteoformation process is mediated by accelerating the apoptosis of mature osteocytes and osteoblasts and the consequent inhibition of osteoblast proliferation. In addition, GC influences the physiological dynamics of parathormone secretion, antagonizes its anabolic action and inhibits the production of insuline-like growth factor (IGF)-1 and testosterone.

Loss of bone mass is evident from the first months of administration, especially in the first year, and mainly affects the trabecular bone, which associates a higher risk of fracture for the vertebral site. Fracture events can occur in 30–50% of patients and are directly related to dose, duration of administration of GCs and patient age.

The assessment of fracture risk in the first six months after initiation of therapy should include an assessment of risk factors and bone mineral density in selected cases and subsequently in accordance with current recommendations. Prevention of GC-induced osteoporosis is done by administering calcium (1000–2000 mg/day) and vitamin D (600–800 IU/day) [37].

7.4 Aseptic osteonecrosis

Aseptic osteonecrosis is the cause of high doses compared to the administration of small, long-term doses, and is rarely seen during prednisone therapy or equivalent of below 20 mg/day [38].

7.5 Myopathy

Cortisone myopathy can occur following the administration of any type of GC and is the consequence of the direct catabolic effect on skeletal muscles. It is clinically evident in the form of proximal muscle weakness, unaccompanied by myalgias or changes in the serum level of muscle enzymes [39].

7.6 Gastrointestinal adverse effects

Glucocorticoids are less toxic to the upper gastrointestinal tract than NSAIDs, but they do raise the risk of adverse gastrointestinal events like gastritis, ulcers and gastrointestinal bleeding. The effect of glucocorticoids on gastrointestinal events is very limited. In addition to evidence of upper gastrointestinal tract morbidity, GCs have been linked to cases of intestinal rupture, diverticular perforation and pancreatitis. In rheumatology, glucocorticoids are commonly used in conjunction with NSAIDs and the two drugs work together to increase the risk of GI side effects [40].

7.7 Ocular adverse effects

Posterior subcapsular cataracts is a well-known side effect of long-term GC therapy. There is no safe dosage for this complication and cataract formation has been documented even with inhaled GC preparations. The use of glucocorticoids has also been linked to cortical cataracts.

Patients taking glucocorticoids can develop cataracts as well as elevated intraocular pressure, which may cause vision problems. The occurrence of frank glaucoma, particularly with low-dose therapy, is uncommon and usually occurs in patients who are genetically predisposed [41].

7.8 Endocrine and metabolic side effects

Exogenous hypercorticism (Cushing's syndrome) is the consequence of long-term high doses and determines the characteristic appearance by redistribution of adipose tissue in the chest, face ("moon facies") and neck ("buffalo bump"), trunk obesity, the appearance of hirsutism, acne, increased appetite, obesity and subsequently the complications represented by osteoporosis, edema, hypertension, growth retardation in children which require dose adjustment or alternative administration - every two days.

Adrenal insufficiency may result from suppression of the hypothalamic–pituitary axis and is directly proportional to dose and duration of administration. High-dose corticosteroids can block the suppression of ACTH release and the rapid onset of adrenal insufficiency in approximately 5 days, lasting up to 4–6 weeks, even at doses of 10–15 mg/day. Restoration of the hypothalamic–pituitary axis usually occurs after 9–12 months. In order to prevent hypercorticism, it is preferred to administer a single morning dose, the use alternative therapy every two days or gradual reduction of the dose.

Changes in glucose metabolism represented by increased blood sugar is a consequence of the stimulation of the process of hepatic neoglucogenesis, hepatic production and storage of glycogen and decreased peripheral glucose utilization. It may cause diabetes or imbalance of pre-existing diabetes. Although the "de novo" onset of diabetes in patients with previously normal glucose levels is relatively rare, the risk is increased in the presence of a family history of diabetes, old age or a history of gestational diabetes.

Changes in lipid metabolism consist in stimulating the lipolysis process and increasing the amount of free fatty acids. The increase in insulin secretion, due to hyperglycemia, will cause a stimulating effect on the lipid metabolism, so that the two concomitant processes, lipolysis/lipogenesis, will cause the reorganization of adipose tissue and the appearance of the characteristic appearance of "lemon on toothpicks".

Protein metabolism is inhibited, except for the hepatic site, with the occurrence of side effects, especially cutaneous, muscular or of the connective tissue [42].

7.9 Cutaneous adverse effects

The most common side effects, even at low doses, are represented by the appearance of bruises and skin atrophy, due to the the acceleration of protein catabolism. In addition, facial erythema, hair fragility, acne and hirsutism may be present [43].

7.10 Neuropsychiatric adverse effects

The spectrum of symptoms is dependent on the dose and duration of administration and may be represented by anxiety, depression, psychosis, delirium, confusion, disorientation, cognitive deficits, sleep disturbances, the appearance of akathisia, usually of mild or moderate intensity. Psychosis is associated with the administration of prednisone at a dose of more than 20 mg/day over a long period of time and may require specific therapy, even under conditions of dose reduction. Behavioral disorders can range from mild euphoria to anxiety or depression in the case of long-term therapy [44].

8. Glucocorticoid therapy in rheumatoid arthritis

In this era of targeted treatments, therapeutic strategies, and comorbidity management in patients with RA, the potential role of GCs in RA is important to consider. Despite the fact that GC therapy was a significant clinical breakthrough for RA in the 1950s, the current focus is on the treatment's drawbacks rather than its benefits.

The aim of RA therapies is to reduce disease activity and achieve clinical remission in the short term, but also to restrict or avoid structural damage and systemic manifestations in the medium term. In RA, GCs have a rather rapid onset of action, which allows time for the DMARDs exert their immunosuppressive effect. Furthermore, GCs are also considered to have a structural impact on the affected joints. However, clinicians tend to use them when in need of rapid symptomatic relief for their RA patients. Thus, the benefit-to-risk ratio of GCs is still uncertain, and their use in RA is still debatable [45].

The use of GCs therapy in RA is regulated by international rheumatology societies such as the European League Against Rheumatism (EULAR) and the American College of Rheumatology (ACR). These societies have formulated recommendations regarding the indications of GC therapy in RA.

The 2015 ACR recommendations for early and established RA state that GC therapy should be used in conjunction with DMARDs at the lowest possible dose and for short periods of time, only in disease flares. Adding GCs when starting a csDMARD, contrary to EULAR guidelines, is dependent on disease activity [46].

The benefit of GCs therapy was emphasized more in recent revisions of the EULAR recommendations for the treatment of early arthritis and RA than in previous versions. Short-term GCs therapy can be taken into consideration in the initial treatment strategy or subsequently if the beneficial effects of the initial strategy have not been considerable, as bridging therapy when a change in DMARD being taken into account. Long-term use of GCs should be discouraged and GCs should be progressively diminished and discontinued, normally by 3 months and only in rare cases by 6 months [47].

These international protocols, taken together, recommend the use of GCs for disease flares and likely at the beginning of a new conventional synthetic DMARD (csDMARD), although specific guidance on dose, duration and length of administration protocols is not yet standardized. A dosage of less than 10 mg/day is considered a low dose in the United States, and GCs could be tapered in less than 3 months, while the European threshold is 7.5 mg/day, and GCs may be administered in conjunction with csDMARDs for up to 6 months total, with the understanding that this duration is mostly expert-driven. Despite these discrepancies, international recommendations stress the effectiveness of GCs while also recommending that they be used at the lowest cumulative dose possible due to the widespread understanding of potential side effects. The doses of GCs are usually expressed in prednisone equivalents in recommendations and studies [48].

In the CareRA trial were included patients with early RA and no negative prognosis signs. Subsequently, they were randomly assigned to one of two treatment arms: Methotrexate associated with GCs in one arm (30 mg/day prednisone tapered to 5 mg/day in 6 weeks) and Methotrexate without the association of GCs in the other arm. At 16 weeks, the patients who received GCs reached Disease Activity Score in 28 Joints (DAS28) remission more compared to the Methotrexate group (65% vs. 47%, p = 0.08). The rates of remission in the Methotrexate and GCs arm were also higher than the Methotrexate-only arm at 1 and 2 years, but not substantially [49].

The results of the BARFOT trial at ten years have been released. The study included 250 patients with early RA. Therapy with csDMARDs alone was compared to csDMARDs plus 7.5 mg/day prednisolone over the course of two years. The patients who recieved GCs demonstrated imporved clinical results at all time points (3, 6, 12, 18, and 24 months). A four-year follow-up analysis showed no variations in the percentage of patients in remission between the two groups. The use of bDMARDs with and without GCs did not vary after ten years. Patients in the BARFOT cohort were included between 1995 and 1999, before the age of biologics, thus the proportion of patients who used a bDMARD was very limited (15% in either group) [50].

In 10 year follow-up of the BeSt study, published in 2016, 508 patients with early active RA were randomly assigned to one of four groups: a pre-determined maintenance care regimen starting with Methotrexate; a group in which sulfasalazine was added to Methotrexate in case of therapy failure; a group following the guidelines of the COBRA study (Sulfasalazine, Methotrexate, and GCs initially at 60 mg/day, then gradually tapered to 7.5 mg/day in 6 weeks) and a group of patients who were administered Methotrexate and Infliximab from the beginning. In the initial study, the protocol in the COBRA trial proved to be more efficient at three months. However, at the 10-year follow-up, almost 50% of patients were in remission regardless of their initial group of randomization, making it difficult to conclude on the long-term beneficial effect of the GC treatment administered in the beginning [51].

The CAPRA-2, the double-blind, placebo controlled trial results were published in 2012. The study included 350 patients with active RA who were randomly assigned 2:1 to receive either modified release (MR) prednisone 5 mg or placebo once daily in the evening in addition to their current RA DMARD therapy for 12 weeks. At week 12, the primary end point was to determine the number of patients who improved by 20% in RA signs and symptoms based on ACR guidelines, respectively the ACR20. Morning pain and stiffness, the 28-joint Disease Activity Score, and health-related quality of life were all evaluated. At week 12, the administration of MR prednisone in conjunction with DMARD therapy proved higher response rates than the administration of placebo plus DMARD in the case of ACR20 (48% vs. 29%) and ACR50 (22% vs. 10%) scores. Overall, low-dose MR prednisone administered in concurrence with DMARD therapy lead to the improvement RA signs and symptoms more quickly and significantly [52].

Results from the SEMIRA trial which included 421 patients with RA divided into two groups: the first group (n = 128) were assigned to the continued prednisone regimen while the second group (n = 131) were assigned to the tapered prednisone regimen. All patients received Tocilizumab for 24 weeks with or without conventional synthetic DMARDs. In patients with low disease activity using Tocilizumab and treatment with GCs for at least 24 weeks, continuous glucocorticoid treatment at a dose of 5 mg per day for 24 weeks provided a safer and better solution than gradual reduction of glucocorticoids, although two-thirds of patients were able to safely reduce their GCs doses [53].

The CAMERA-II study's post-trial follow-up results were released in 2017. The study group included 236 patients with RA. CAMERA-II compared the administration of Methotrexate plus 10 mg/day prednisone for two years to a Methotrexate and placebo group. After two years of therapy, disease activity decreased more in the Methotrexate-GCs arm than in the Methotrexate-placebo arm on average, but the variations seen in the first months continued to fade with time. Patients in the Methotrexate-GCs group had initiated a biological DMARD slightly less often than those in the Methotrexate-placebo group (31% vs. 50%) during the follow-up analysis, with a median follow-up of about 6.6 years.

Given these findings, there is little question whether GCs will reduce disease activity in RA patients, at least in the short term. It's impossible to say if the therapeutic advantage of GCs will last in the short and long term. Because of their toxicity and limited structural impact, GCs should never be used alone and should always be combined with DMARDs [54].

9. Glucocorticoid therapy in connective tissue diseases

9.1 Systemic lupus erythematosus

Systemic lupus erythematosus (SLE) is one of the most severe autoimmune rheumatic diseases, with multisystemic involvement, with frequent flares and an increased risk of death. The treatment of SLE is guided by organ damage, but most often it is represented by a combination of hydroxychloroquine - the gold standard in SLE - and variable doses of corticosteroids depending on the severity of the visceral damage and often in combination with immunosuppressants agents. Early and aggressive treatment in SLE is essential for the prevention of organ damage, the 2019 EULAR recommendations for the treatment of SLE supporting both the prevention of organ damage and the improvement of patients' quality of life and their long-term survival [55]. Achieving remission or low disease activity is another important goal in SLE management. Complete remission, defined as the absence of disease activity in the absence of treatment with CS or immunosuppressant, is rare [56].

For the patients with active disease, CS in variable doses, in combination with hydroxychloroquine and sometimes with immunosuppressants agents, still represent the optimal management of SLE. Besides the anti-inflammatory and immunosuppressive effects, the side effects of CS are well known, most of them are time and dose dependent: osteoporosis, osteonecrosis, cataract, hyperglycemia or coronary heart disease. Although they produce a rapid reduction in symptoms and the recommendation is to reduce the doses ≤7.5 mg/day equivalent to prednisone, or discontinued therapy, some studies have shown adverse effects even at minimal doses of cortisone [57]. Thus, it is recommended the administration of intravenous methylprednisolone pulse therapy (250–1000 mg/day for 3 consecutive days) depending on the body weight, during acute flares and also the early initiation of immunosuppressive agents, both having the role of initiating a lower oral dose, as well as a faster reduction of CS doses [58].

For skin damage, the first therapeutic line, in addition to avoiding exposure to UV radiation, is represented by topical CS. Oral CS can also be used, depending on the degree of skin damage [59].

Cardiovascular involvement in SLE is one of the main causes of death, due by both kidney damage, that can cause cardiovascular and cerebrovascular disorders, but also by the increased risk of developing atherosclerosis, a consequence of both chronic inflammation and the additional risk of CS [60]. In a study of a group of 175 women with SLE, Manzi et al. identified the presence of carotid plaques in 40% of them, which correlated with the cumulative dose of prednisone and with the duration of therapy. Similar results were recorded in other studies that showed the relationship between prednisone and weight gain, blood pressure or a high serum cholesterol, correlation with sudden death or demonstration of subclinical atheromatosis in 45% of a group of 78 Italian patients with SLE [61].

The risk of infections in SLE is caused by the activity of the disease, by severe leukopenia and by the administration of high doses of CS in association with immunosuppressants agents. The results of a 2009 case–control study showed that the risk of severe infections was higher in the group of patients with prednisone 7.5 mg/day vs. those who received a median dose of 2.5 mg/day thus demonstrating that the risk of developing infections increases by 12% for every mg/day.

In summary, CSs has an importnat role in SLE, but side effects, often dependent on dose and duration of administration, should not be overlooked. Therefore, intravenous pulsetherapy with methylprednisolone is preferred, with consequent faster reduction of oral doses, and also the combination of antimalarials and immunosuppressive agents in the therapeutic regimen [62].

9.2 Systemic scleroderma

In systemic scleroderma, the use of CS is controversial, due to the lack of response of vasculopathy and fibrosis to CS, and due to the increased risk of developing scleroderma renal crisis. Itchy skin, arthralgia and myalgia in early and very early diffuse cutaneous systemic sclerosis have been shown to respond to low doses of CS, thus suggesting an inflammatory skin component in these stages, characterized by perivascular and tissue infiltrates with monocytes, macrophages and CD4 + lymphocytes. Thus, the effects of CS can be beneficial in these stages, before the appearance of irreversible fibrotic changes. Also, doses of CS can be used in interstitial lung disease related to systemic scleroderma. Asthenia in scleroderma may have a good response to CS administration, although there are no studies on this. Another benefit in patients with scleroderma is increased appetite, although it is well known that it is considered an adverse effect of corticosteroids, in patients with scleroderma it may be considered a benefit [63].

One of the most serious complications of systemic scleroderma is *scleroderma renal crisis* (SRC). Risk factors for its occurrence are: diffuse cutaneous forms, positivity of anti-RNA polymerase III antibodies and the use of CS. The mechanisms by which CS can trigger SRC are given in particular by vasoconstriction caused by the stimulation of endogenous and exogenous catecholamines by cortisol. Thus, there is a reduction in the production of prostaglandins by the endothelium, thus causing vasospasm. There is a decrease in juxtaglomerular perfusion by reducing the secretion of prostaglandin E2 (PGE2) with consecutive vasoconstriction of renal arterioles [64].

There are many studies that have shown that CS administration is a major risk factor for the development of SRC. Steen and Medsger in 1998 demonstrated in a case–control study that 36% of a group of 110 patients with SRC had received doses >15 mg/day equivalent of prednisone in the last 6 months [65]. Similar results were recorded in another studies in France - 60% of 50 patients with SRC had received CS with a mean duration of 2.65 months before the onset of SRC, respectively 59% of 64 patients with SRC in a study in UK [66, 67]. Montanelli et al. showed a 1.5% increased risk of developing SRC for each mg/day of prednisone administration [68]. The International Renal Crisis Survey has shown an increased risk of death of 4% for each mg/day of prednisone administration [69].

In contrast, there were open-label studies, but performed on a small number of patients with early difuse cutaneous systemic sclerosis, who not report SRC at low doses of CS.

CS are still ones of the most used therapies in *interstitial lung disease* in scleroderma. In 2018, EUSTAR showed that 60% of patients with interstitial lung disease were treated with CS, regardless of whether or not scleroderma was in the early stages of the disease [70].

For *cardiomyopathy* in scleroderma, doses of CS <15 mg/day of the equivalent of prednisone, alone or in combination with cyclophosphamide, have been shown to have beneficial effects.

In conclusion, GC can be indicated in the early and very early stages of systemic scerosis, when there is mainly inflammation, without fibrosis, indicated for skin or musculoskeletal damage, but should be used with caution, to very low-dose and a short time duration, to avoid CRS [71].

9.3 Inflammatory myopathies

CS are the first-line medication in polymiositis (PM) and dermatomyositis (DM). Patients with myositis and lung interstitial disease require high doses of CS, either 1 g methylprednisolone/day in pulse therapy - 3 consecutive days with subsequent oral follow-up or 60 mg/day for 3–4 months with monitoring clinical and biological parameters. Dose reduction is generally slow, usually with 5 mg/week. Some patients may relapse at dose reduction in these situation an immunosuppressive agent such as methotrexate or azathioprine may be associated; if muscle damage decreases with decreasing CS doses, but skin involvement persists, hydroxychloroquine may be associated [72]. High doses of CS, as well as long duration of administration, can cause glucocorticoid-induced myositis, so this condition must be differentiated by the relaps with pain and muscle weakness. If the increase in CS doses worsens the symptoms means it is glucocorticoid-induced myositis. Although some studies show that high-dose CS improves the prognosis in both PM and DM, another study has shown that mortality and morbidity in both poly- and dermatomyositis are elevated even at high doses of CS [73].

9.4 Sjőgren's syndrome

Sjőgren's syndrome is an autoimmune disease, characterized by the presence of anti-Ro and anti-La antibodies, a mononuclear focal infiltrate of the exocrine glands and whose main manifestations are xerostomia and xerophthalmia. Oral CS administration in primary Sjőgren syndrome has been shown to correlate with decreased proinflammatory cytokine levels, but with increased anti-Ro52 and anti-Ro-60 antibodies levels [74]. The same study did not show an increase in salivary volume after CS administration, in contrast to the study by Miyawaki et al. who demonstrated that there was a significant increase in salivary volume upon initiation of

CS treatment, but with a reduction after 48 months of follow-up. Haldorsen et al. showed in a study that neither the use of hydroxychloroquine nor CS influenced salivary production [75].

Regarding the effects of CS in lowering autoantibodies levels, a small study in a group of 20 patients with Sjögren syndrome who received low-dose of CS had significantly reduced levels of both anti-Ro/SSA and anti- La/SSB antibodies, an effect that maintained a 48-month follow-up in 5 patients from the group, compared to the study of Reksten et al. which showed an increase in anti-Ro52 and anti-Ro-60 antibodies levels in patients with primary Sjogren syndrome treated with CS [76].

For *eye involvement* in Sjögren syndrome, topical CS can also be used, but for a short period of time and with caution due to the increased risk of cataract, glaucoma or local infections especially during the exacerbation of sicca keratoconjunctivitis.

For *extraglandular involvement*, low doses of CS may be used in combination with hydroxychloroquine for musculoskeletal damage, arthralgias, myalgia or high doses or pulsetherapy of methylprednisolon in glomerulonephritis.

In *neurological impairment* in Sjögren syndrome, such as acute transverse myelitis, the current treatment is an association of pulsetherapy of methylprednisolone with cyclophosphamide.

The role of CS alone or in combination with other immunosuppressive agents in the management of connective-tissue diseases is unquestionable, but it should be used with caution, in the lowest effective dose and for as short a period of time as possible to minimize the adverse effects [77].

10. Glucocorticoid therapy in systemic vasculitis

In the case active *large vessel vasculitis*, EULAR recommendations from 2018 are to initiate therapy with GCs in high doses (40–60 mg/day equivalent of prednisone), followed by tapering of the dose in 2–3 months to 15–20 mg/day, if the patients is in remission, and to 7.5–10 mg/day at 6 months. Subsequently, after more than 1 year of CS therapy, it is recommended to maintain a dose of ≤5 mg/day for giant cell arteritis and ≤ 10 mg/day for Takayasu arteritis and cease GCs therapy at 18–24 months. Therefore, for patients with no eye damage, the administration of 1 mg/kg/day of prednisone ≤60 mg/day causes a significant improvement in symptoms in 24–48 hours and a significant reduction of the inflammatory tests.

Decreases in dose reduction of corticosteroids are common in large vessel vasculitis, so in the case of minor relapses it is recommended to increase the dose of glucocorticoids to the last effective dose and in case of a major relapse it is recommended to increase the dose to 40–60 mg/day.

In case of acute blindness or amaurosis fugax in giant cell arteritis, it is recommended to administer pulse therapy with 500 mg - 1 g/day of intravenous methylprednisolone for 1–3 days followed by the administration of oral GCs, at a dose of 1 mg/kg/day, less than 60 mg/day, but the ocular damage is rarely reversible and loss of visual acuity may persist despite initiation of GC treatment in approximately 10% of patients [78].

The treatment of *polymyalgia rheumatica* is based on the 2015 EULAR/ACR recommendations. It is recommended to use the lowest effective GC dose of 12.5–25 mg/day equivalent of prednisone. It is necessary to individualize the dose reduction according to the clinical and biological profile of each patient. The following dose reduction principles are recommended:

- initial decrease - to 10 mg/day equivalent of prednisone in 4–8 weeks;

- relapse therapy - increasing the dose of glucocorticoids to the dose before relapse and gradually decreasing it in 4–8 weeks until the dose at which the relapse occurred;

- dose reduction in case of remission - the dose of prednisone is reduced by 1 mg every 4 weeks until discontinuation of therapy, as long as remission is maintained [79].

The therapeutic approach in *polyarteritis nodosa* patients with a five factor score (FFS) of 0 is the use of GCs in monotherapy. The doses used are pulse therapy with 500–1000 mg methylprednisolone/day for 3–5 days followed by 1 mg/kg/day of oral equivalent of prednisone in order to obtain remission, with the subsequent progressive decrease of doses. In the presence of severe organ damage, cyclophosphamide in combination with GCs is recommended in patients with FFS ≥ 1. The recommended doses are 2 mg/kgc/day orally or the administration of intravenous therapy of 600 mg/m^2 at intervals of 2–4 weeks, for 3–6 months [80].

In *ANCA-associated vasculitis*, the EULAR/ERA-EDTA recommendations state that GCs should be administered in doses of 1 mg/kg/day of equivalent of prednisone or in pulse therapy with methylprednisolone 1 g/day for 3 consecutive days to induce remission associated with cyclophosphamide or rituximab. The target is to reduce the dose to 7.5–10 mg/day equivalent of prednisone after 3 months of treatment. To induce remission in limited forms without severe organ damage, the use of methotrexate in doses of 20–25 mg/week or mycophenolate mofetil in doses of 2–3 g/day in combination with GCs is recommended [81].

In the case of *Behçet's disease*, the treatment is based on the EULAR recommendations of 2018. Thus, arterial lesions benefit from treatment with GCs in high doses, pulse therapy with 1 g/day methylprednisolone for 3 days, followed by of 1 mg/kg/day equivalent of prednisone and intravenous cyclophosphamide in monthly courses, if no surgery is required.

In the case of neurological manifestations, depending on the severity of the clinical manifestations, pulse therapy with GC in doses of 1 g/day is administered for 7 days, followed by oral prednisone at doses of 1 mg/kgc/day for one month and slow dose reduction by 5–10 mg every 10–15 days.

Ocular involvement benefits from topical treatment with GC or for the rapid suppression of episodes of acute inflammation of high doses of systemic GC. In the case of refractory cutaneous and mucosal manifestations, low doses of oral GC may be used [82].

11. Corticosteroids in local injections for inflammatory rheumatic disease

Injection therapy using corticosteroids in the local treatment of multiple musculoskeletal disorders has been used with success for already more than 70 years, nevertheless, only a few studies of its application in joint and periarticular lesions based on expert opinion and outcome measures in rheumatology define efficacy and compare local injection of corticosteroids with other treatments.

Several controversies regarding the local mechanism of action in rheumatic conditions, dosing regimen, volume, which type of steroid, injection technique, optimal schedule of injecting or for how long, blind or ultrasound guided placement of injection have arose as most of these aspects are non-standardized.

A decade after the first systemic use of steroid drugs, Hollander, in the USA reported the first documented use of hydrocortisone intra-articular injections for arthritis [83].

The rationale for injecting corticosteroids has become apparent after analyzing side effects generated by their systemic administration. Several mechanisms of action and pharmacological effects are proposed when injected into the joints and soft tissues, but the premise is that injecting insoluble corticosteroid suspensions in limited quantities, in contact with inflamed tissues will determine the up taking of the active drug by the synovial cells, before being absorbed in lesser amount in the blood and cleared, thus reducing the systemic effects [84].

The major effect when used in intra and periarticular injections is that of suppressing inflammation in inflammatory rheumatic diseases such as rheumatoid arthritis, ankylosing spondylitis, psoriatic arthritis or gout. As in systemic administration they exert these effects mostly by modulating the transcription of multiple genes, acting by binding on nuclear steroid receptors in order to regulate the rate of synthesis of mRNA and proteins, subsequently reducing the production of pro-inflammatory cytokines [85]. Administration of steroids can be done intra-articular, in the synovial sheath of tendons for tenosynovitis, for dactilitis, bursitis or entesitis.

Another indication for injecting local steroids is suppression of inflammatory flares in degenerative joint disease, although benefits over disadvantages are still subject of debate. The risk of infection, Charcot-like arthritis, aseptic osteonecrosis or cartilage loss through altered protein synthesis may overweight the favorable response of pain and inflammation. Still, studies sustain major improvement of pain and inflammation in osteoarthritis of the knee after local injection of corticosteroids (triamcinolone hexacetonide) compared to placebo, persistent for up to six weeks after administration. Improvement may be due also to the benefits of joint aspiration of pathological fluid. A review of intra-articular corticosteroid for knee osteoarthritis in terms of pain, physical function, quality of life and safety, that searched the Cochrane Central Register of Controlled Trials (CENTRAL), MEDLINE, and EMBASE (from inception to 3 February 2015), including 27 trials with 1767 participants identified that intra-articular corticosteroids appeared to be more beneficial in pain reduction than control interventions (SMD -0.40, 95% CI -0.58 to −0.22). In terms of follow up benefits were moderate at 1 to 2 weeks after end of treatment (SMD -0.48, 95% CI -0.70 to −0.27), small to moderate at 4 to 6 weeks (SMD -0.41, 95% CI -0.61 to −0.21), small at 13 weeks (SMD -0.22, 95% CI -0.44 to 0.00), and no evidence of an effect at 26 weeks (SMD -0.07, 95% CI -0.25 to 0.11). Corticosteroids have showed to be more effective also in function improvement than control interventions (SMD -0.33, 95% CI -0.56 to - 0.09), while no evidence has been proved of an effect of corticosteroids on quality of life compared to control (SMD -0.01, 95% CI -0.30 to 0.28, I2 = 0%). Patients with corticosteroid injections were 11% less likely to experience adverse events, 67% less likely to withdraw because of adverse events, and 27% less likely to experience any serious adverse event, but confidence intervals were wide and included the null effect.

There is little evidence to support another rationale for using local corticosteroids such as the clivage of the inflammatory damage – repair – damage cycle that mentaines a continuous low-grade inflammatory response by inhibiting tissue repair and scarr formation in favor of adhesion formation [86].

Several studies support a direct protective effect on the cartilage metabolism through promotion of articular surfactant production and not related to the anti-inflammatory effect of corticosteroids [87].

Corticosteroids used for intra-articular injections differ in terms of potency and time of action, solubility playing an important role in choosing the best drug according to indication. The most frequently used corticosteroid for local administration are illustrated in **Table 2**.

Local side effects of injectable corticosteroids may occur when injected too often or when the volume and dose are not adjusted to the anatomy of the joint, as well as when injecting the enthesis of the tendons with large quantities of corticosteroids.

Joint infection is one of the most severe local adverse effects that is most likely to occur between 4 days and 3 weeks after the procedure, usually in a immunocompromised patient or with high risk of infections such as diabetics, or patients with joint arthroplasties or intravenous lines [88]. After injecting periarticular soft tissues local infection and osteomyelitis may be suggested by increasing pain, local swelling, fever or systemic signs of infection.

Synovial and *subcutaneous tissue irritation* or *postinjection flare* usually happens after soft tissue injection and is caused by the rapid intracellular ingestion of the microcrystalline steroid ester, more frequent after methylprednisolone with pain and swelling that may mimic and should be differentiated from sepsis. Pain, swelling, limited range of motion and stiffness suggests transient synovitis after joint injection. Not only the steroid itself may cause a postinjection flare, but preservatives such as parabens may be incriminated in te appearance of a local irritative reaction [89].

Steroid arthropathy is mostly linked to frecquent number of corticosteroid injections with reports of Charcot-like joint distruction after osteoarthritic hip injection, with conflicting evidence over the risk due to corticosteroids or rather to the disease progression itself [90]. Most reports support the rather chondroprotective effect of steroids than chondrolitic, while repeating steroid injections no sooner than 3 months seems to be safe over a period of 2 years [91].

Prolonged bleedeng at the procedural site or *bruising* may occur in patients taking anticoagulants, vasodilators, aspirin or NSAIDs with significant antiplatelet activity. Anticoagulation within a therapeutical INR does not contraindicate joint injection of corticosteroids.

Skin depigmentation is mostly due to injecting superficial lesions or when drug refluates back through the needle tract after retraction, mostly in dark-skinned patients. Of more interest is *local atrophy* of skin and subcutaneous tissue that may appear as late as one to four months after injection bu. usually dissapears in six months to two years [92]. Also, *steroid "chalk" or "paste" deposits* after substance flocculation may be detected through surgery at the level of previously injected joints and tendons [93], as well as *soft tissue calcifications*.

Injecting corticosteroids into tendons associated with *tendon rupture or atrophy* is widely accepted although not well supported from studies [94]. Adjusting the dose and the volume injected, avoiding injecting enthesis or using peppering technique may minimise the risks (**Figure 1**).

Duration of action	Drug	Equivalent of prednisone
Short-acting	Hydrocortisone acetate	5 mg
Intermediate-acting	Methylprednisolone acetate	50 mg
	Triamcinolone acetonide	50 mg
	Triamcinolone hexacetonide	25 mg
Long-acting	Betamethasone sodium phosphate	50 mg

Table 2.
Corticosteroids frequently used for local administration.

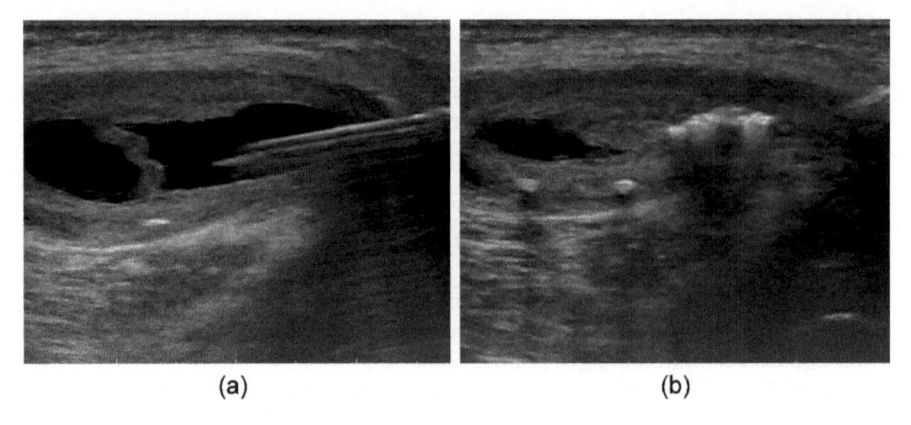

Figure 1.
(A) Aspiration of a Baker cyst guided by ultrasound. (B) Hyperechoic images consistant of steroid deposits after injection.

More rare side effects are linked mostly to the injecting technique or expertise, such as nerve damage when needling a nerve, transient paresis or needle fracture [95].

12. Conclusions

Corticosteroids still remain the anchor drugs in therapy strategies in inflammatory rheumatic diseases even though new drugs such as biologic or targeted synthetic molecules have emerged in the past years. In diseases such as systemic vasculitis, some of the connective tissue diseases such as SLE and poly/dermatomyositis GCs are considered the first-line therapy. Thus, it is of great importance to acknowledge the use of GCs in rheumatology.

Conflict of interest

The authors declare no conflict of interest.

Author details

Anca Emanuela Mușetescu[1], Cristina Criveanu[1], Anca Bobircă[2], Alesandra Florescu[3*], Ana-Maria Bumbea[4] and Florin Bobircă[5]

1 Department of Rheumatology, University of Medicine and Pharmacy of Craiova, Craiova, Romania

2 Department of Internal Medicine and Rheumatology, Carol Davila University of Medicine and Pharmacy, Bucharest, Romania

3 Department of Rheumatology, Emergency Clinical County Hospital of Craiova, Craiova, Romania

4 Department of Medical Rehabilitation, University of Medicine and Pharmacy of Craiova, Craiova, Romania

5 Department of General Surgery, Carol Davila University of Medicine and Pharmacy, Bucharest, Romania

*Address all correspondence to: alesandracioroianu@yahoo.com

IntechOpen

© 2021 The Author(s). Licensee IntechOpen. This chapter is distributed under the terms of the Creative Commons Attribution License (http://creativecommons.org/licenses/by/3.0), which permits unrestricted use, distribution, and reproduction in any medium, provided the original work is properly cited.

References

[1] Kapugi M, Cunningham K. Corticosteroids. Orthop Nurs. 2019;38:336-339. DOI: 10.1097/NOR.0000000000000595

[2] Hardy R, Rabbitt EH, Filer A, Emery P, Hewison M, Stewart PM, Gittoes NJ, Buckley CD, Raza K, Cooper MS. Local and systemic glucocorticoid metabolism in inflammatory arthritis. Ann Rheum Dis. 2008;67:1204-10. DOI: 10.1136/ard.2008.090662.

[3] Munck A, Naray-Fejes-Toth A. Glucocorticoids and stress: permissive and suppressive actions. Ann NY Acad Sci. 1994; 746:115-30. DOI: 10.1111/j.1749-6632.1994.tb39221.x

[4] Burns CM. The History of Cortisone Discovery and Development. Rheum Dis Clin North Am. 2016;42:1-14. DOI: 10.1016/j.rdc.2015.08.001.

[5] Benedek TG. History of the development of corticosteroid therapy. Clin Exp Rheumatol. 2011;29:5-12.

[6] Hench PS, Kendall EC, Slocumb CH, Polley HF. The effect of a hormone of the adrenal cortex (17-hydroxy-11-dehydrocorticosterone: compound E) and of pituitary adrenocortical hormone in arthritis: preliminary report. Ann Rheum Dis. 1949;8:97-104. DOI: 10.1136/ard.8.2.97.

[7] Wijdicks EFM, Rooke TW, Hunder GG, Dacy MD. Cortisone in Popular Culture: Roueché, Ray, and Hench. Mayo Clin Proc Innov Qual Outcomes. 2019;3:215-220. DOI: 10.1016/j.mayocpiqo.2019.04.003.

[8] Warner ME. Witness to a miracle: The initial cortisone trial: An interview with Richard Freyberg, M.D. Mayo Clin Proc. 2001;76: 529-532.

[9] Hench PS. The reversibility of certain rheumatic and nonrheumatic conditions by the use of cortisone or of the pituitary adrenocorticotropic hormone. Ann Intern Med. 1952; 36: 1-38.

[10] Freyberg RH, Traeger CT, Adams CH, Kuscu T, Wainerdi H, Bonomo I. Effectiveness of cortisone administered orally. Science. 1950;112:429. DOI: 10.1126/science.112.2911.429.

[11] Ruiz-Irastorza G, Ugarte A, Ruiz-Arruza I, Khamashta M. Seventy years after Hench's Nobel prize: revisiting the use of glucocorticoids in systemic lupus erythematosus. Lupus. 2020;29:1155-1167. DOI: 10.1177/0961203320930099.

[12] Boland EW: The treatment of rheumatoid arthritis with adrenocorticosteroids and their synthetic analogues: an appraisal of certain developments of the past decade. Ann NY Acad Sci. 1959; 82: 887-901.

[13] Hardy RS, Raza K., Cooper MS. Therapeutic glucocorticoids: mechanisms of actions in rheumatic diseases. Nat Rev Rheumatol. 2020.16:133-144. DOI: 10.1038/s41584-020-0371-y.

[14] Strehl C, Ehlers L, Gaber T, Buttgereit F. Glucocorticoids-All-Rounders Tackling the Versatile Players of the Immune System. Front Immunol. 2019;24;10:1744. DOI: 10.3389/fimmu.2019.01744.

[15] Franco LM, Gadkari M, Howe KN, Sun J, Kardava L, Kumar P, Kumari S, Hu Z, Fraser IDC, Moir S, Tsang JS, Germain RN. Immune regulation by glucocorticoids can be linked to cell type-dependent transcriptional responses. J Exp Med. 2019;216:384-406. DOI: 10.1084/jem.20180595.

[16] Croxtall JD, van Hal PT, Choudhury Q, Gilroy DW, Flower RJ. Different glucocorticoids vary in their genomic and non-genomic mechanism of action in A549 cells. Br J Pharmacol.

[17] Stahn C, Buttgereit F. Genomic and nongenomic effects of glucocorticoids. Nat Clin Pract Rheumatol. 2008;4:525-533. DOI: 10.1038/ncprheum0898.

[18] Belvisi MG, Wicks SL, Battram CH, Bottoms SE, Redford JE, Woodman P, Brown TJ, Webber SE, Foster ML. Therapeutic benefit of a dissociated glucocorticoid and the relevance of in vitro separation of transrepression from transactivation activity. J Immunol. 2001;166(3):1975-82. DOI: 10.4049/jimmunol.166.3.1975.

[19] Altonsy MO, Sasse SK, Phang TL, Gerber AN. Context-dependent cooperation between nuclear factor κB (NF-κB) and the glucocorticoid receptor at a TNFAIP3 intronic enhancer: a mechanism to maintain negative feedback control of inflammation. J Biol Chem. 2014;289:8231-8239. DOI: 10.1074/jbc.M113.545178.

[20] Almawi WY, Melemedjian OK. Molecular mechanisms of glucocorticoid antiproliferative effects: antagonism of transcription factor activity by glucocorticoid receptor. J Leukoc Biol. 2002;71:9-15.

[21] Herold MJ, McPherson KG, Reichardt HM. Glucocorticoids in T cell apoptosis and function. Cell Mol Life Sci. 2006;63:60-72. DOI: 10.1007/s00018-005-5390-y.

[22] Rook GA. Glucocorticoids and immune function. Baillieres Best Pract Res Clin Endocrinol Metab. 1999;13:567-81. DOI: 10.1053/beem.1999.0044.

[23] van de Garde MD, Martinez FO, Melgert BN, Hylkema MN, Jonkers RE, Hamann J. Chronic exposure to glucocorticoids shapes gene expression and modulates innate and adaptive activation pathways in macrophages with distinct changes in leukocyte attraction. J Immunol. 2014;192:1196-208. DOI: 10.4049/jimmunol.1302138.

[24] Alam J, Jantan I, Bukhari SNA. Rheumatoid arthritis: Recent advances on its etiology, role of cytokines and pharmacotherapy. Biomed Pharmacother. 2017;92:615-633. DOI: 10.1016/j.biopha.2017.05.055.

[25] Shimba A, Ikuta K. Glucocorticoids Regulate Circadian Rhythm of Innate and Adaptive Immunity. Front Immunol. 2020;11:2143. DOI: 10.3389/fimmu.2020.02143.

[26] Adcock IM, Mumby S. Glucocorticoids. Handb Exp Pharmacol. 2017;237:171-196. DOI: 10.1007/164_2016_98.

[27] Rose SP. Cell-adhesion molecules, glucocorticoids and long-term-memory formation. Trends Neurosci. 1995;18:502-506. DOI: 10.1016/0166-2236(95)92774-k.

[28] Czock D, Keller F, Rasche FM, Häussler U. Pharmacokinetics and pharmacodynamics of systemically administered glucocorticoids. Clin Pharmacokinet. 2005;44:61-98. DOI: 10.2165/00003088-200544010-00003.

[29] Strehl C, Spies CM, Buttgereit F. Pharmacodynamics of glucocorticoids. Clin Exp Rheumatol. 2011;29(5 Suppl 68):S13-8.

[30] Jacobs JW, Bijlsma JW. Glucocorticoids in rheumatology: indications and routes of administration. Clin Exp Rheumatol. 2011;29(5 Suppl 68):S81-4.

[31] Buttgereit, F. Views on glucocorticoid therapy in rheumatology: the age of convergence. Nat Rev Rheumatol. 2020;16:239-246. DOI: 10.1038/s41584-020-0370-z.

[32] Strehl C, Bijlsma JW, de Wit M, Boers M, Caeyers N, Cutolo M, Dasgupta B, Dixon WG, Geenen R, Huizinga TW, Kent A, de Thurah AL,

Listing J, Mariette X, Ray DW, Scherer HU, Seror R, Spies CM, Tarp S, Wiek D, Winthrop KL, Buttgereit F. Defining conditions where long-term glucocorticoid treatment has an acceptably low level of harm to facilitate implementation of existing recommendations: viewpoints from an EULAR task force. Ann Rheum Dis. 2016;75:952-957. DOI: 10.1136/annrheumdis-2015-208916.

[33] Youssef J, Novosad SA, Winthrop KL. Infection Risk and Safety of Corticosteroid Use. Rheum Dis Clin North Am. 2016;42:157-176. DOI: 10.1016/j.rdc.2015.08.004.

[34] Ng MK, Celermajer DS. Glucocorticoid treatment and cardiovascular disease. Heart. 2004;90:829-30. DOI: 10.1136/hrt.2003.031492.

[35] Shen JZ, Young MJ. Corticosteroids, heart failure, and hypertension: a role for immune cells? Endocrinology. 2012;153:5692-700. DOI: 10.1210/en.2012-1780.

[36] Chotiyarnwong P, McCloskey EV. Pathogenesis of glucocorticoid-induced osteoporosis and options for treatment. Nat Rev Endocrinol. 2020;16:437-447. DOI: 10.1038/s41574-020-0341-0.

[37] Briot K, Roux C. Glucocorticoid-induced osteoporosis. RMD Open. 2015;1(1):e000014. DOI: 10.1136/rmdopen-2014-000014.

[38] Lai SW, Lin CL, Liao KF. Evaluating the association between avascular necrosis of femoral head and oral corticosteroids use in Taiwan. Medicine (Baltimore). 2020;99(3):e18585. DOI: 10.1097/MD.0000000000018585.

[39] Sun LY, Chu XL. Acute myopathy following intra-muscular injection of compound betamethasone: A case report. Medicine (Baltimore). 2017; 96(34):e7474. DOI: 10.1097/MD.0000000000007474.

[40] Narum S, Westergren T, Klemp M. Corticosteroids and risk of gastrointestinal bleeding: a systematic review and meta-analysis. BMJ Open. 2014;**4**:e004587. DOI: 10.1136/bmjopen-2013-004587.

[41] Phulke S, Kaushik S, Kaur S, Pandav SS. Steroid-induced Glaucoma: An Avoidable Irreversible Blindness. J Curr Glaucoma Pract. 2017;11:67-72. doi: 10.5005/jp-journals-l0028-1226.

[42] van der Goes MC, Jacobs JW, Bijlsma JW. The value of glucocorticoid co-therapy in different rheumatic diseases--positive and adverse effects. Arthritis Res Ther. 2014;16 Suppl 2(Suppl 2):S2. DOI: 10.1186/ar4686.

[43] Kannan S, Khan W, Bharadwarj A, Rathore BS, Khosla PP. Corticosteroid-induced cutaneous changes: A cross-sectional study. Indian J Pharmacol. 2015;47:696-8. DOI: 10.4103/0253-7613.169583.

[44] Warrington TP, Bostwick JM. Psychiatric adverse effects of corticosteroids. Mayo Clin Proc. 2006;81:1361-1367. DOI: 10.4065/81.10.1361.

[45] Buttgereit F, Bijlsma JW. Glucocorticoids in rheumatoid arthritis: the picture is shaping up. Ann Rheum Dis. 2017;76:1785-1787. doi: 10.1136/annrheumdis-2017-211187.

[46] Black RJ, Lester S, Buchbinder R, Barrett C, Lassere M, March L, Whittle S, Hill CL. Factors associated with oral glucocorticoid use in patients with rheumatoid arthritis: a drug use study from a prospective national biologics registry. Arthritis Res Ther. 2017;19:253. DOI: 10.1186/s13075-017-1461-3.

[47] Hua C, Buttgereit F, Combe B. Glucocorticoids in rheumatoid arthritis: current status and future studies. RMD Open. 2020;**6**:e000536. DOI: 10.1136/rmdopen-2017-000536.

[48] Chatzidionysiou K, Emamikia S, Nam J, Ramiro S, Smolen J, van der Heijde D, Dougados M, Bijlsma J, Burmester G, Scholte M, van Vollenhoven R, Landewé R. Efficacy of glucocorticoids, conventional and targeted synthetic disease-modifying antirheumatic drugs: a systematic literature review informing the 2016 update of the EULAR recommendations for the management of rheumatoid arthritis. Ann Rheum Dis. 2017;76:1102-1107. DOI: 10.1136/annrheumdis-2016-210711.

[49] Verschueren P, De Cock D, Corluy L, Joos R, Langenaken C, Taelman V, Raeman F, Ravelingien I, Vandevyvere K, Lenaerts J, Geens E, Geusens P, Vanhoof J, Durnez A, Remans J, Vander Cruyssen B, Van Essche E, Sileghem A, De Brabanter G, Joly J, Meyfroidt S, Van der Elst K, Westhovens R. Effectiveness of methotrexate with step-down glucocorticoid remission induction (COBRA Slim) versus other intensive treatment strategies for early rheumatoid arthritis in a treat-to-target approach: 1-year results of CareRA, a randomised pragmatic open-label superiority trial. Ann Rheum Dis. 2017;76:511-520. DOI: 10.1136/annrheumdis-2016-209212.

[50] Hafström I, Albertsson K, Boonen A, van der Heijde D, Landewé R, Svensson B; BARFOT Study Group. Remission achieved after 2 years treatment with low-dose prednisolone in addition to disease-modifying anti-rheumatic drugs in early rheumatoid arthritis is associated with reduced joint destruction still present after 4 years: an open 2-year continuation study. Ann Rheum Dis. 2009;68:508-13. DOI: 10.1136/ard.2008.087833.

[51] Markusse IM, Akdemir G, Dirven L, Goekoop-Ruiterman YP, van Groenendael JH, Han KH, Molenaar TH, Le Cessie S, Lems WF, van der Lubbe PA, Kerstens PJ, Peeters AJ, Ronday HK, de Sonnaville PB, Speyer I, Stijnen T, Ten Wolde S, Huizinga TW, Allaart CF. Long-Term Outcomes of Patients With Recent-Onset Rheumatoid Arthritis After 10 Years of Tight Controlled Treatment: A Randomized Trial. Ann Intern Med. 2016;164:523-31. DOI: 10.7326/M15-0919.

[52] Buttgereit F, Mehta D, Kirwan J, Szechinski J, Boers M, Alten RE, Supronik J, Szombati I, Romer U, Witte S, Saag KG. Low-dose prednisone chronotherapy for rheumatoid arthritis: a randomised clinical trial (CAPRA-2). Ann Rheum Dis. 2013;72:204-10. DOI: 10.1136/annrheumdis-2011-201067.

[53] Burmester GR, Buttgereit F, Bernasconi C, Álvaro-Gracia JM, Castro N, Dougados M, Gabay C, van Laar JM, Nebesky JM, Pethoe-Schramm A, Salvarani C, Donath MY, John MR, SEMIRA collaborators. Continuing versus tapering glucocorticoids after achievement of low disease activity or remission in rheumatoid arthritis (SEMIRA): a double-blind, multicentre, randomised controlled trial. Lancet. 2020;396(10246):267-276. DOI: 10.1016/s0140-6736(20)30636-x.

[54] Safy M, Jacobs J, IJff ND, Bijlsma J, van Laar JM, de Hair M; Society for Rheumatology Research Utrecht (SRU). Long-term outcome is better when a methotrexate-based treatment strategy is combined with 10 mg prednisone daily: follow-up after the second Computer-Assisted Management in Early Rheumatoid Arthritis trial. Ann Rheum Dis. 2017;76:1432-1435. DOI: 10.1136/annrheumdis-2016-210647.

[55] Fanouriakis A, Kostopoulou M, Alunno A, Aringer M, Bajema I, Boletis JN, Cervera R, Doria A, Gordon C, Govoni M, Houssiau F, Jayne D, Kouloumas M, Kuhn A, Larsen JL, Lerstrøm K, Moroni G, Mosca M, Schneider M, Smolen JS, Svenungsson E, Tesar V, Tincani A, Troldborg A, van Vollenhoven R, Wenzel J, Bertsias G, Boumpas DT. 2019 update of the EULAR

recommendations for the management of systemic lupus erythematosus. Ann Rheum Dis. 2019;78:736-745. DOI: 10.1136/annrheumdis-2019-215089.

[56] Steiman AJ, Urowitz MB, Ibañez D, Papneja A, Gladman DD. Prolonged clinical remission in patients with systemic lupus erythematosus. J Rheumatol. 2014;41:1808-1816. DOI: 10.3899/jrheum.131137.

[57] Tsang-A-Sjoe MW, Bultink IE, Heslinga M, Voskuyl AE. Both prolonged remission and Lupus Low Disease Activity State are associated with reduced damage accrual in systemic lupus erythematosus. Rheumatology (Oxford). 2017;56:121-128. DOI: 10.1093/rheumatology/kew377.

[58] Al Sawah S, Zhang X, Zhu B, Magder LS, Foster SA, Iikuni N, Petri M. Effect of corticosteroid use by dose on the risk of developing organ damage over time in systemic lupus erythematosus-the Hopkins Lupus Cohort. Lupus Sci Med. 2015;2:e000066. DOI: 10.1136/lupus-2014-000066.

[59] Thamer M, Hernán MA, Zhang Y, Cotter D, Petri M. Prednisone, lupus activity, and permanent organ damage. J Rheumatol. 2009;36:560-4. DOI: 10.3899/jrheum.080828.

[60] Ruiz-Arruza I, Lozano J, Cabezas-Rodriguez I, Medina JA, Ugarte A, Erdozain JG, Ruiz-Irastorza G. Restrictive Use of Oral Glucocorticoids in Systemic Lupus Erythematosus and Prevention of Damage Without Worsening Long-Term Disease Control: An Observational Study. Arthritis Care Res (Hoboken). 2018;70:582-591. DOI: 10.1002/acr.23322.

[61] Manzi S, Selzer F, Sutton-Tyrrell K, Fitzgerald SG, Rairie JE, Tracy RP, Kuller LH. Prevalence and risk factors of carotid plaque in women with systemic lupus erythematosus. Arthritis Rheum. 1999;42:51-60. DOI: 10.1002/1529-0131(199901)42:1<51::AID-ANR7>3.0.CO;2-D.

[62] Ruiz-Irastorza G, Danza A, Khamashta M. Glucocorticoid use and abuse in SLE. Rheumatology (Oxford). 2012;51:1145-1153. DOI 10.1093/rheumatology/ker410.

[63] Chairta P, Nicolaou P, Christodoulou K. Genomic and genetic studies of systemic sclerosis: A systematic review. Hum Immunol. 2017;78:153-165. DOI: 10.1016/j.humimm.2016.10.017.

[64] Hamaguchi Y, Kodera M, Matsushita T, Hasegawa M, Inaba Y, Usuda T, Kuwana M, Takehara K, Fujimoto M. Clinical and immunologic predictors of scleroderma renal crisis in Japanese systemic sclerosis patients with anti-RNA polymerase III autoantibodies. Arthritis Rheumatol. 2015;67:1045-1052. DOI: 10.1002/art.38994.

[65] Steen VD, Medsger TA Jr. Case-control study of corticosteroids and other drugs that either precipitate or protect from the development of scleroderma renal crisis. Arthritis Rheum. 1998;41:1613-1619. DOI: 10.1002/1529-0131(199809)41:9<1613::AID-ART11>3.0.CO;2-O.

[66] Teixeira L, Mouthon L, Mahr A, Berezné A, Agard C, Mehrenberger M, Noël LH, Trolliet P, Frances C, Cabane J, Guillevin L; Group Français de Recherche sur le Sclérodermie (GFRS). Mortality and risk factors of scleroderma renal crisis: a French retrospective study of 50 patients. Ann Rheum Dis. 2008;67:110-6. DOI: 10.1136/ard.2006.066985.

[67] Penn H, Howie AJ, Kingdon EJ, Bunn CC, Stratton RJ, Black CM, Burns A, Denton CP. Scleroderma renal crisis: patient characteristics and long-term outcomes. QJM. 2007;100:485-494. doi: 10.1093/qjmed/hcm052.

[68] Montanelli G, Beretta L, Santaniello A, Scorza R. Effect of

dihydropyridine calcium channel blockers and glucocorticoids on the prevention and development of scleroderma renal crisis in an Italian case series. Clin Exp Rheumatol. 2013;31(2 Suppl 76):135-139.

[69] Hudson M, Baron M, Tatibouet S, Furst DE, Khanna D; International Scleroderma Renal Crisis Study Investigators. Exposure to ACE inhibitors prior to the onset of scleroderma renal crisis-results from the International Scleroderma Renal Crisis Survey. Semin Arthritis Rheum. 2014;43:666-672. DOI: 10.1016/j.semarthrit.2013.09.008.

[70] Adler S, Huscher D, Siegert E, Allanore Y, Czirják L, DelGaldo F, Denton CP, Distler O, Frerix M, Matucci-Cerinic M, Mueller-Ladner U, Tarner IH, Valentini G, Walker UA, Villiger PM, Riemekasten G; EUSTAR co-workers on behalf of the DeSScipher project research group within the EUSTAR network. Systemic sclerosis associated interstitial lung disease - individualized immunosuppressive therapy and course of lung function: results of the EUSTAR group. Arthritis Res Ther. 2018;20(1):17. DOI: 10.1186/s13075-018-1517-z.

[71] Bissell LA, Anderson M, Burgess M, Chakravarty K, Coghlan G, Dumitru RB, Graham L, Ong V, Pauling JD, Plein S, Schlosshan D, Woolfson P, Buch MH. Consensus best practice pathway of the UK Systemic Sclerosis Study group: management of cardiac disease in systemic sclerosis. Rheumatology (Oxford). 2017;56:912-921. DOI: 10.1093/rheumatology/kew488.

[72] Cordeiro AC, Isenberg DA. Treatment of inflammatory myopathies. Postgrad Med J. 2006;82:417-24. DOI: 10.1136/pgmj.2005.038455.

[73] Mușetescu AE, Ciurea PL, Cioroianu A, Florescu LM, Bumbea AM, Pîrșcoveanu DFV, Brăila AD. Extensive Bone Infarctions - an Unexpected Consequence of Corticosteroid Treatment in Idiopathic Polymiositis. Rev. Chim.(Bucharets). 2018; 69: 1122-1124.

[74] Reksten TR, Brokstad KA, Jonsson R, Brun JG, Jonsson MV. Implications of long-term medication of oral steroids and antimalarial drugs in primary Sjögren's syndrome. Int Immunopharmacol. 2011;11:2125-2129. DOI: 10.1016/j.intimp.2011.09.006.

[75] Miyawaki S, Nishiyama S, Matoba K. Efficacy of low-dose prednisolone maintenance for saliva production and serological abnormalities in patients with primary Sjögren's syndrome. Intern Med. 1999;38:938-943. DOI: 10.2169/internalmedicine.38.938.

[76] Aragona P, Rania L, Roszkowska AM, Spinella R, Postorino E, Puzzolo D, Micali A. Effects of amino acids enriched tears substitutes on the cornea of patients with dysfunctional tear syndrome. Acta Ophthalmol. 2013;91:e437-44. doi: 10.1111/aos.12134.

[77] Ramos-Casals M, Brito-Zerón P, Bombardieri S, Bootsma H, De Vita S, Dörner T, Fisher BA, Gottenberg JE, Hernandez-Molina G, Kocher A, Kostov B, Kruize AA, Mandl T, Ng WF, Retamozo S, Seror R, Shoenfeld Y, Sisó-Almirall A, Tzioufas AG, Vitali C, Bowman S, Mariette X; EULAR-Sjögren Syndrome Task Force Group. EULAR recommendations for the management of Sjögren's syndrome with topical and systemic therapies. Ann Rheum Dis. 2020;79:3-18.DOI:10.1136/annrheumdis-2019-216114.

[78] Hellmich B, Agueda A, Monti S, Buttgereit F, de Boysson H, Brouwer E, Cassie R, Cid MC, Dasgupta B, Dejaco C, Hatemi G, Hollinger N, Mahr A, Mollan SP, Mukhtyar C, Ponte C, Salvarani C, Sivakumar R, Tian X, Tomasson G, Turesson C, Schmidt W, Villiger PM, Watts R, Young C, Luqmani RA. 2018 Update of the EULAR recommendations for the

management of large vessel vasculitis. Ann Rheum Dis. 2020;79:19-30. DOI: 10.1136/annrheumdis-2019-215672.

[79] Dejaco C, Singh YP, Perel P, Hutchings A, Camellino D, Mackie S, Abril A, Bachta A, Balint P, Barraclough K, Bianconi L, Buttgereit F, Carsons S, Ching D, Cid M, Cimmino M, Diamantopoulos A, Docken W, Duftner C, Fashanu B, Gilbert K, Hildreth P, Hollywood J, Jayne D, Lima M, Maharaj A, Mallen C, Martinez-Taboada V, Maz M, Merry S, Miller J, Mori S, Neill L, Nordborg E, Nott J, Padbury H, Pease C, Salvarani C, Schirmer M, Schmidt W, Spiera R, Tronnier D, Wagner A, Whitlock M, Matteson EL, Dasgupta B; European League Against Rheumatism; American College of Rheumatology. 2015 recommendations for the management of polymyalgia rheumatica: a European League Against Rheumatism/American College of Rheumatology collaborative initiative. Arthritis Rheumatol. 2015; 67:2569-80. DOI: 10.1002/art.39333.

[80] Ozen S. The changing face of polyarteritis nodosa and necrotizing vasculitis. Nat Rev Rheumatol. 2017;13:381-386. DOI: 10.1038/nrrheum.2017.68.

[81] Yates M, Watts RA, Bajema IM, Cid MC, Crestani B, Hauser T, Hellmich B, Holle JU, Laudien M, Little MA, Luqmani RA, Mahr A, Merkel PA, Mills J, Mooney J, Segelmark M, Tesar V, Westman K, Vaglio A, Yalçındağ N, Jayne DR, Mukhtyar C. EULAR/ERA-EDTA recommendations for the management of ANCA-associated vasculitis. Ann Rheum Dis. 2016;75:1583-94. DOI: 10.1136/annrheumdis-2016-209133.

[82] Hatemi G, Christensen R, Bang D, Bodaghi B, Celik AF, Fortune F, Gaudric J, Gul A, Kötter I, Leccese P, Mahr A, Moots R, Ozguler Y, Richter J, Saadoun D, Salvarani C, Scuderi F, Sfikakis PP, Siva A, Stanford M, Tugal-Tutkun I, West R, Yurdakul S, Olivieri I, Yazici H. 2018 update of the EULAR recommendations for the management of Behçet's syndrome. Ann Rheum Dis. 2018;77:808-818. DOI: 10.1136/annrheumdis-2018-213225.

[83] Hollander JL, Brown EM, Jester RA et al. Hydrocortisone and cortisone injected into arthritic joints; comparative effects of a use of hydrocortisone as a local anti-arthritis agent. Journal of the American Medical Association. 1951;147:1629-1635. DOI: 10.1001/jama.1951.03670340019005.

[84] Derendorf H, Möllmann H, Grüner A, Haack D, Gyselby G. Pharmacokinetics and pharmacodynamics of glucocorticoid suspensions after intra-articular administration. Clin Pharmacol Ther. 1986;39:313-317. DOI: 10.1038/clpt.1986.45.

[85] Creamer P. Intraarticular corticosteroid injections in osteoarthritis: do they work and if so how? Annals of Rheumatic Diseases 1997;56:634-636. DOI: 10.1136/ard.56.11.634

[86] Jüni P, Hari R, Rutjes AW, Fischer R, Silletta MG, Reichenbach S, da Costa BR. Intra-articular corticosteroid for knee osteoarthritis. Cochrane Database Syst Rev. 2015;(10):CD005328. DOI: 10.1002/14651858.CD005328.pub3.

[87] Larsson E, Erlandsson Harris H, Larsson A, Månsson B, Saxne T, Klareskog L. Corticosteroid treatment of experimental arthritis retards cartilage destruction as determined by histology and serum COMP. Rheumatology (Oxford). 2004;43:428-434. DOI: 10.1093/rheumatology/keh073.

[88] Ryan MJ, Kavanagh R, Wall PG, Hazleman BI. Bacterial joint infections in England and Whales: analysis of bacterial isolates over a four year period. British Journal of Rheumatology. 1997; 36:370-373. DOI: 10.1093/rheumatology/36.3.370.

[89] Gray RG, Gottlib NI. Basic science and pathology: intra-articular corticosteroids, an updated assessement Clinical Orthopaedics and Related Research 1982;177:235-263. DOI: 10.1093/rheumatology/36.3.370.

[90] Jones A, Doherty M. Intra-articular steroid injections are effective in OA but there are no clinical predictors of response. Annals of the Rheumatic Diseases. 1996;55:829-832. DOI: 10.1136/ard.55.11.829.

[91] Kirwan JR, Rankin E. Intra-articular therapy in osteoarthritis. Baillieres Clinical Rheumatology. 1997;11:769-794. DOI: 10.1016/s0950-3579(97)80009-x.

[92] Birrer RB. Aspiration and corticosteroid injection. Physiology and Sports Medicine 1992;20:57-71.

[93] Kumar N, Newman R. Complications of intra- and peri-articular steroid injections. British Journal of General Practice. 1999;49:465-466.

[94] Cooper C, Kirwan JR. Risks of corticosteroid therapy. Clinical Rheumatology 1990;19:305-332.

[95] Fredberg U. Local corticosteroid injection in sport: review of literature and guidelines for treatment. Scandinavian Journal of Medicine and Science in Sport 1997;7:131-139. DOI: 10.1111/j.1600-0838.1997.tb00129.x.

Chapter 3

Corticosteroids in Otorhinolaryngology

Magdalena B. Skarzynska and Piotr H. Skarzynski

Abstract

This paper aims to present the role of the therapy of corticosteroids in otorhinolaryngological diseases such as Meniere's disease, partial deafness, sudden sensorineural hearing loss, and tinnitus. The effectiveness of treatment depends on many factors, for instance, the duration of the therapy, occurrence or not of adverse reactions, especially in those patients with additional risk factors as comorbidities. Additionally, the optimal way of administration has been widely discussed.

Keywords: corticosteroids, cochlear implantation, partial deafness treatment, tinnitus, Meniere's disease, administration, sudden sensorineural hearing loss, cochlear implant, otorhinolaryngology

1. Introduction

Corticosteroids play an important role in the pharmacological treatment in different otorhinolaryngological disorders such as Sudden Sensorineural Hearing Loss (SSNHL), Meniere's Disease (MD), Tinnitus and as a supportive treatment in the different ENT (ear-nose-throat) surgery procedures, including cochlear implantation (CI). The effectiveness of therapy of corticosteroids in otorhinolaryngology depends on many different factors. The main are: the duration of the therapy, occurrence or not of adverse reactions, especially in those patients with additional risk factors as comorbidities. A widely discussed challenge among ENT scientists is the optimal way of administration of corticosteroids – local or systemic – due to the different pharmacokinetic and pharmacodynamic properties of corticosteroids. One of these is the effective delivery way of a drug to its place of action, because of the presence of blood-labyrinth barrier (BLB) and the inaccessibility due to the inner ear.

2. Pharmacokinetics of corticosteroids and delivery to the inner ear

From a pharmacokinetic point of view, the inner ear can be considered to be made up of multiple fluid compartments in hydrostatic balance (maintained by the blood-labyrinth barrier). The pharmacokinetic process is helpfully described by the acronym LADME (L – liberation; A – absorption; D – distribution; M – metabolism; E – elimination). The first step – liberation – means that the drug (or its carrier) must be water-soluble, so it can easily be carried in the blood [1].

The next pharmacokinetic step is absorption and depends on lipophilicity and the solubility of the drug [1]. Only a few drugs can be used effectively in otorhinolaryngological practice due to the difficulty of achieving sufficient concentrations in the inner ear [2]. Two groups of drugs are commonly used in clinical practice: aminoglycosides (mainly gentamicin) in the pharmacotherapy of Meniere's disease, and corticosteroids (dexamethasone, triamcinolone) in pharmacotherapy for idiopathic sudden sensorineural hearing loss and other cases of acute hearing loss [3].

The distribution process depends on many different factors as a route of administration, mode of administration, single or repeated administration, dose, ionic composition, pH, and osmolarity. The elimination of a drug from the body (its clearance rate) depends on the same set of chemical and physical properties. A key factor here is the protein binding of the drug: the greater the protein binding of the drug, the longer its therapeutic activity. The finite binding between the protein and the drug molecule allows the drug to gradually liberate.

As far as, the inner ear drug delivery strategies are concerned, three routes of administration are possible: systemic (intravenous, oral), intratympanic, and intracochlear [4]. Systemic administration of glucocorticoids is reasonable due to pharmacological properties such as the lipophilic nature of glucocorticoids and vascularity of the middle ear mucosa [5]. Blood labyrinth barrier (BLB) and round window membrane (RWM) are two main challenges in delivering drugs to the inner ear. Blood labyrinth barrier is the most important barrier that separates the inner ear from systemic blood circulation and, as a result, maintains the microhomeostasis in the inner ear. This barrier protects also the integrity of the inner ear due to the presence of efflux pumps system such as MRP-1 (multidrug resistance-related protein-1) and P-glycoprotein. The tight junctions permit to penetrate only small lipid-soluble molecules. The concentration of corticoids in the perilymph increase when the osmotic agent (e.g. glycerol) is added. RWM is a soft tissue barrier which role is to separate the inner ear from the middle ear and it is permeable to low molecular weight molecules such as corticoids. Generally and despite the adverse effects, systemic delivery (oral, intravenous, intramuscular routes) is still considered as the most convenient method of drug administration and the first-line approach in the treatment of inner ear disorders [4]. Additionally, both oral and intravenous route of administration is complied with the characteristic of medical products used in this study.

The intratympanic route of administration may be performed via injection or perfusion to the middle ear. The drawbacks of intratympanic delivery of drug include such barriers as: anatomic barriers (RWM), loss of drug in the middle ear cavity through the Eustachian tube and the pharmacokinetic profile of administrated drugs is unknown or variable [6, 7]. As a result, the number and percentage of drugs that may enter the inner ear are relatively low.

The intracochlear route of drug delivery can bypass the middle ear and allows drug to get the direct place of action. Although this strategy seems to be more risky in terms of deafness, according to the observations of surgical procedures which include perforation and significant manipulations [8]. Currently, there is no available safe and effective technique for intracochlear drug administration not only in terms of medical device but also in terms of appropriate drug formulation [4].

In the summary, the inner ear is a very subtle and complicated organ from anatomical and physiological point of view. Hearing loss may be one of the most dangerous and severe adverse effects in the inner ear caused by novel drug delivery systems. All routes of drug administration should be carefully examined and considered.

3. Corticosteroids in cochlear implantation

In a study published in 2018, Plontke, Götze, Rahne & Liebau compared the effects of dexamethasone with saline (in a guinea pig model). Both substances were administrated intravenously 60 minutes before implantation. The conclusion was that dexamethasone could reduce scarring in the hook region or near the electrode tip, but they did not see any relation between dexamethasone and reduction of fibrosis relating to cochleostomy. At the same time, in vitro studies have shown a correlation between reduction (loss) of auditory cells after exposure to tumor necrosis factor-alpha and dexamethasone-releasing polymer (used to coat the CI electrode carrier) [9–12].

Cochlear implantation is a golden standard for patients who suffer from severe to profound hearing loss. The preservation of hearing in patients who underwent cochlear implantation depends, in the first place, on surgical technique, and in the second place, on the selecting of the appropriate electrode. The pharmacological treatment, such as administration of corticosteroids in different periods of cochlear implantation, is the third important factor [6, 7]. Insertion of the frequency-specific electrode array into the cochlea is a delicate operation and requires a very careful surgical technique. Even with the utmost care, however, it is difficult not to cause some tissue damage, especially in cases of partial deafness where there are still some partially functioning hair cells. In this situation, the use of corticosteroids (local or systemic) is important: these drugs can reduce oxidative stress, inflammatory reaction, and the apoptosis of hair cells due to insertion damage. A major challenge in effectively delivering pharmacological agents to the cochlea is its physical inaccessibility and the presence of a blood-labyrinth barrier. These factors are especially apt for patients suffering partial deafness, where the hair cells at the apex of the cochlea (responsible for receiving low frequencies) are anatomically remote.

4. Corticosteroids in Meniere's disease

Symptoms of Meniere's disease are defined as recurring episodes of spontaneous, usually rotational vertigo, sensorineural hearing loss, tinnitus, and a feeling of fullness or pressure in the affected ear for up to decades. The disease can be unilateral or bilateral. The diagnosis of the disease is made based on the symptoms present, however, it is sometimes difficult to make, because the diagnosis should exclude other diseases that exhibit symptoms similar to Meniere's disease, such as dizziness of other origins, occurring independently with hearing loss and tinnitus, and may react differently to treatment (e.g. mild positional vertigo, acute labyrinthitis, migraine) and to hearing neuronal. The disease most often affects adults between the ages of 30 and 60. It is estimated to affect 50-200/100,000 cases annually in Europe [13].

Meniere's disease is associated with anatomical changes in the inner ear: the so-called endolymphatic swellings. The volume of the endolymph, which fills the endolymphatic labyrinth, increases while the volume of the perilymph, which surrounds the endolymphatic labyrinth and fills the bony labyrinth, decreases. However, swelling occurs in many other conditions associated with hearing loss and there is no known cause of this condition. Specific disorders associated with swelling (such as temporal bone fracture, syphilis, end-stage otosclerosis, and auditory nerve neuroma) may produce symptoms similar to those of Meniere's disease. Meniere's disease initially progresses but changes unpredictably. It is difficult to distinguish natural resolution from treatment effects, as dizziness resolves in 57% of patients after 2 years and 71% after 8 years with the disease [13, 14].

The primary goal of pharmacotherapy is to reduce the frequency, duration, and severity of vertigo attacks. The secondary goals are to stop the progression of hearing loss and to reduce the occurrence of tinnitus. Unfortunately, no medication can currently slow or stop the progression of hearing loss or stop tinnitus.

The use of corticosteroids (CS) in the treatment of MD has been implicated because of the presence of autoimmune disorders in the course of the disease, and the role of the innate immune system and inflammation in the pathophysiology of MD. Studies have revealed the presence of glucocorticoid receptors in the inner ear. The action of corticosteroids in the course of MD is based on their anti-inflammatory and immunosuppressive effects, as well as regulation of inner ear homeostasis [15–17]. The treatment of MD includes the use of oral dexamethasone or methylprednisolone to reduce vomiting and vestibular symptoms, particularly in cases of marked hearing loss, but there are no RCTs showing any long-term benefit of steroids in MD [16]. When administered by intratympanic injection, CS achieve higher concentrations in the inner ear compared to systemic administration, with fewer systemic side effects [16, 18]. Substances administered intratympanically include dexamethasone and methylprednisolone, one that triamcinolone is also a therapeutic option. Studies have shown that methylprednisolone gives higher concentrations in the endolymph and perilymph than dexamethasone, but the latter drug may be more effective because it is more rapidly absorbed by endocytosis into the vascular striatum and surrounding tissues, where it acts intracellularly [19, 20]. Several retrospective/prospective control placebo or non-control studies have assessed intratympanic administration of CS, with varying remission results [14, 21–31]. An RCT study by Garduño-Anaya et al. showed that inner ear perfusion with dexamethasone (4 mg/ml) in a group of patients with unilateral Meniere's disease, demonstrated 82% complete control of vertigo compared to placebo (57%) [25]. In a subsequent study using an extended-release form of intrathecally administered dexamethasone, the form was shown to reduce the number of definitive days with dizziness, the severity of dizziness, and the mean daily number of dizziness compared with placebo at month 3 after drug administration [32, 33]. The systematic review combined these two RCTs with the Garduño-Anaya study with a total of 220 patients. The authors of this new review conclude that there is still no solid confirmation that ITC has a positive effect in MD [16, 34]. Although the results of some studies support the conclusion that high-dose steroid is effective in treating MD, the optimal treatment protocol has not yet been properly established. In addition, the development of an appropriate protocol to confirm the unequivocal efficacy of CS in MD is difficult because there is considerable variability in patients' symptoms and over time, as well as a group of patients in the population who do not respond to CS treatment [14, 35, 36].

5. Corticosteroids in sudden sensorineural hearing loss

Sudden sensorineural hearing loss (SSNHL) is a syndrome that develops rapidly, with hearing loss progressing over 72 hours, hearing loss observed by at least 30 dB at 3 consecutive frequencies on tonal audiometry. It is considered an otologic emergency requiring immediate diagnosis and treatment. The disease can occur at any age; however, it most commonly affects patients 65 years of age or older. The annual incidence of SSNHL is 5-27 per 100,000. According to clinical guidelines for the treatment of SSNHL, systemic CS is recommended as initial therapy and intratympanic CS is recommended as salvage therapy, but the latter is increasingly used as first-line therapy. In addition, pharmacotherapeutic models combining both routes of administration are appropriate [37]. Because of the risk of catastrophic consequences of permanent severe hearing loss, administration of CS should be done as soon as possible, allowing the greatest improvement to be seen within the first two weeks, but continuing therapy for an additional 6 weeks. The mechanism of action of CS is still uncertain, but its effect is possible due to its ability to reduce inflammation and swelling [38]. Treatment uses a 7-14 day series of oral high doses of prednisone — (1 mg/kg/d max. 60 mg/d), methylprednisolone — 48 mg/d or dexamethasone at 10 mg/d, despite possible side effects [39]. Treatment by intratympanic injection has efficacy equivalent to systemic administration with the benefit of reducing the proportion of adverse reactions occurring after systemic administration as well as when oral administration is not possible or contraindicated [40–46]. In addition, Crane et al. also looked at the efficacy of intratympanically administered steroids against intratympanically administered steroids as initial therapy and showed no overall superiority of intratympanically administered steroids over systemic steroids, with the single exception of the Battaglia et al. study, which showed an advantage of using intratympanically administered CS without or in combination with systemic versus using systemic CS alone [39, 47, 48]. The frequency of IT steroid administration also varies widely in different studies, and may be self-administered by the patient through a pressure equalization tube several times a day to physician administration from once a day to once a week or less frequently. Intratympanic treatments include: Dexamethasone (DEX) at a dose of 1.5-2 mg, Methylprednisolone at a dose of 25-40 mg or Triamcinolone Acetonide at a dose of 40 mg [39, 49]. Alexander et al. in their retrospective study comparing the response to two different doses of DEX demonstrated that in patients receiving DEX the preferred unit dose of 24 mg/mL dexamethasone in a series of three doses over a 1-3 week period in a variable dose from 0.5-1 mL dependent on anatomical [50]. Given the available literature, corticosteroids may not be used to treat SSNHL in every case. However, for a patient with severe to profound SSNHL, corticosteroid treatment is one of the few treatment options for which there are any data indicating efficacy, although even these data are somewhat inconclusive.

6. Corticosteroids in tinnitus

Tinnitus is the perception of sound without an external stimulus. This symptom can occur alone or with other disorders such as hearing loss. Subjective tinnitus is the most common form of tinnitus, and globally, it can be detected in almost 10% of the general population, and approximately 20% of adults with tinnitus require clinical intervention. The most common site of subjective tinnitus is the cochlea, but other auditory pathways may also be responsible. Tinnitus can occur on one or both sides of the head and can be perceived as coming from inside the head or from outside the head, and is most common with coexisting sensorineural hearing loss. The presence of tinnitus has been shown to affect a patient's quality of life (QOL) in a variety of ways, ranging from a mild deterioration in QOL to severe anxiety, depression, and extreme life-altering events, including the presence of active suicidal thoughts. Many different treatments for tinnitus have been described, including: tinnitus correction, tinnitus masking, biofeedback therapy, and various pharmacological treatments; however, these treatments have limited effectiveness. The most common pharmacological treatments include intratympanic administration of aminoglycoside antibiotics and steroids. CS are used in the treatment of tinnitus due to their anti-inflammatory and electrolyte-modifying effects. According to the available literature, the therapeutic effect of drugs administered intratympanically occurs by diffusion through the round window, the annular ligament of the oval window, the capillaries, or through the lymphatic system of the inner ear. However, the effectiveness of intratympanic therapy in the treatment of tinnitus remains limited [51, 52]. The American Academy of Otolaryngology guidelines provide detailed patient management criteria and outline pharmacologic treatment options for patients with varying levels of confidence and recommendations. These recommendations address the treatment of tinnitus with intratympanic steroid injection and present models of pharmacotherapy using dexamethasone or methylprednisolone with or without concomitant therapy. Based on the RCTs cited in the guideline, steroids are not recommended for the treatment of vertigo because no treatment has shown a better response compared to placebo [51, 53–56]. However, the scientific literature reports positive effects of steroid treatment of tinnitus, indicating that there is still a need for a broad investigation of the contribution of steroids to the treatment of tinnitus. In a study by Yaner et al. a statistically significant parameter score was obtained indicating positive treatment effects with intratympanic dexamethasone versus placebo [52]. Subsequently, a study by Shim et al. indicates the positivity of intratympanic injection of dexamethasone as an adjunctive treatment for tinnitus in patients treated with alprazolam [57]. The positive aspects of adding a steroid to therapy were confirmed by Albu and Chirtes, in their RCT. The addition of dexamethasone to melatonin therapy had a statistically significant effect on reducing tinnitus compared to melatonin alone [58]. Most articles on the subject conclude that intratympanic steroid injections are effective mostly in patients with acute tinnitus and mostly show no effect in those with chronic tinnitus [52, 59]. The studies presented here primarily utilize dexamethasone as the drug administered to the patient; however, it is not the only substance used. The literature reports that intratympanic administration of methylprednisolone has also been studied; however, data detailing the effectiveness of each substance in the treatment of tinnitus remains scarce. Only She et al. in their study compared the efficacy of two types of steroids together with oral carbamazepine, where they found no statistically significant differences indicating the benefit of using individual substances [55]. In opposition to these results indicating an effect of methylprednisolone, is a study by Topak et al. who in their placebo-controlled RCT showed that the steroid had no benefit in the treatment of subjective tinnitus of cochlear origin refractory to treatment [56]. For the treatment of tinnitus, the effect of subcutaneously administered triamcinolone acetonide was analyzed in an RCT by Diao et al. However, it has no obvious benefit over placebo for subjective tinnitus [60]. The use of steroids in the treatment of tinnitus is widespread, as illustrated by the multitude of studies that have been conducted, but there is still a need for strong evidence to support or exclude their use in the treatment of subjective tinnitus.

7. Practical aspects of the administration of corticosteroids in cochlear implantation

The main aim of the present study was to compare the hearing preservation levels of partial deafness patients following cochlear implant surgery when two different procedures for administrating dexamethasone (or dexamethasone and prednisone) were used with different cochlear implants. Patients enrolled in the study suffered severe to profound hearing loss and were classified according to the Skarżyński Partial Deafness Treatment (PDT) classification scheme [61] into two groups: PDT-EC (Partial Deafness Treatment – Electrical Stimulation) or PDT-EAS (Partial Deafness Treatment – Electro-Acoustic Stimulation) (**Figure 1**).

The inclusion and exclusion criteria were in accordance with the consensus of the international HEARRING group on hearing preservation in cochlear implantation. Study eligibility criteria were participants ≥18 years of age with a cochlear duct ≥27.1 mm (measured by computerized tomography), with:

- hearing levels in the range of 10-120 dB HL at frequencies of 125–250 Hz;

- hearing levels of 35–120 dB HL at frequencies of 500–1,000 Hz;

- hearing levels of 75–120 dB HL at frequencies of 2,000–8,000 Hz.

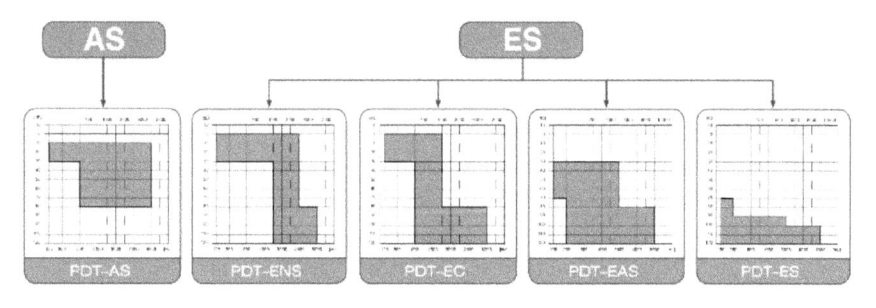

Corticosteroids in Otorhinolaryngology
DOI: http://dx.doi.org/10.5772/intechopen.98636

Figure 1.
Partial deafness treatment groups for cochlear implantation. ENS – Electro-natural stimulation; EC – Electrical complement; EAS – Electrical-acoustic stimulation; ES – Electrical stimulation.

Exclusion criteria included suffering from a severe disease for which steroid treatment could worsen the patient's condition or where might be possible interactions between the patient's medications and steroids. Non-parametric tests were used due to differences in the number of participants between subgroups, the small number of participants in the study, and the violation of normal distribution of pure tone audiometry results [62].

Patients who were enrolled in this prospective study were divided into 3 subgroups. Patients from the first subgroup underwent intravenous (IV) steroid therapy (**Figure 2**). For patients in the first subgroup, dexamethasone was administrated intravenously (0.1 mg per kg of body mass) 30 minutes before the cochlear implant surgery. The same dose was administered every 12 hours for 3 consecutive days (6 doses). The dexamethasone used in this study was supplied in ampoules of a 2 mL solution (4 mg/mL). Before injection, the sterile contents of the ampoule were diluted with isotonic sodium chloride solution. To standardize corticosteroid delivery, the IV route of administration was chosen.

Patients from the second subgroup underwent combined oral and IV corticosteroid therapy (prolonged steroid therapy) following cochlear implantation (**Figure 3**). Prednisone was administered orally at a dose of 1 mg per kg of body mass 3 days before surgery. Then 30 minutes before the implantation surgery, dexamethasone at a dose of 0.1 mg per kg of body mass was administered IV (as with the first group). During the next 3 days, prednisone was administered orally (1 mg of prednisone per kg body mass). After this time, the dose was reduced by about 10 mg per day until it reached zero. To investigate the effects of prolonged steroid administration, we chose to compare the IV and oral administration routes.

The third subgroup was a control group. Patients enrolled in this group underwent a standard cochlear implantation procedure without steroid treatment.

The primary outcome variables were mean hearing thresholds averaged across all 11 measured frequencies (0.125–8 kHz). A secondary outcome variable was hearing preservation (HP). HP was calculated by comparing hearing thresholds in the 1-year postoperative period with preoperative hearing thresholds according to the HP formula in section 3.3 and classified into one of three levels: minimal, partial, or complete hearing preservation.

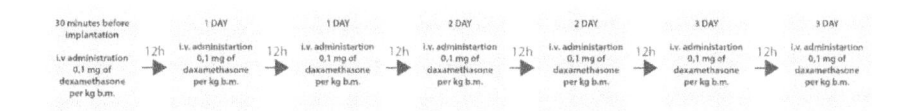

Figure 2.
Scheme of steroid administration in the first subgroup of patients.

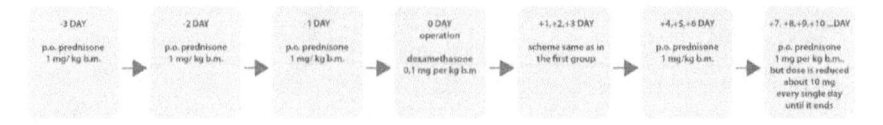

Figure 3.
Scheme of administration of steroids in the second subgroup of patients.

The clinical effect of administered substances was evaluated by pure tone audiometry over six different periods: before cochlear implant surgery (first point), at the activation of the audio processor (second point), and 1 (third point), 6 (fourth point), 9 (fifth point), and 12 months (sixth point) after activation of the audio processor. There were three different periods in Medel and Oticon implants: the preoperatively period (the first point), at the activation of the audio processor (the second point), and 12 months after activation of the audio processor (the third point). Non-parametric tests were used due to the differences in size between each of the groups. Statistical analysis was performed using IBM SPSS software v.24.0.

The mean hearing preservation rate (HP) was 52.1% (SD = 36.7) in patients with standard steroid therapy, 71.4% (SD = 22.7) in patients with prolonged steroid therapy, and 22.1% (SD = 33.9) in the control group. The smallest variation in hearing preservation rate was observed in patients with prolonged steroid therapy.

Data concerning hearing preservation converted to three categories (minimal, partial, complete). HP is defined as follows (**Figure 4**).

In this equation, PTApre is the pure tone average measured preoperatively, PTApost is the pure tone average measured postoperatively, and PTAmax is the maximum sound intensity generated by a standard audiometer (usually 120 dB HL) and HP is the degree of hearing preservation as a percentage [63].

Preoperatively, there were no statistically significant differences in hearing thresholds between patients in each of the three subgroups, including the control group, which means that all study participants had similar hearing levels in the preoperative period.

Deterioration of mean hearing thresholds in pure-tone audiometry (PTA) was observed from the first follow-up interval, which is at the time of sound processor activation. Statistically significant differences were observed between the second sub-group (combined steroid treatment: prednisone + dexamethasone) and the control group: patients in the second study subgroup have obtained better PTA results in low frequencies than the control group. A similar observation was made in the measurements performed at 1, 6, 9, and 12 months after activation of the sound processor – patients who underwent the combined (prolonged) glucocorticoid treatment had more stable hearing thresholds in all follow-up periods (**Figures 5–8**).

The rate of hearing preservation was calculated following the formula based on the PTA measurements performed 12 months after implant activation and preoperatively. The results were then divided into three groups according to the HP classification: minimal HP, partial HP, and complete HP. The smallest variability

$$HP = \left(1 - \frac{PTApost - PTApre}{PTAmax - PTApre}\right) * 100 \; [\%]$$

Figure 4.
Hearing preservation formula.

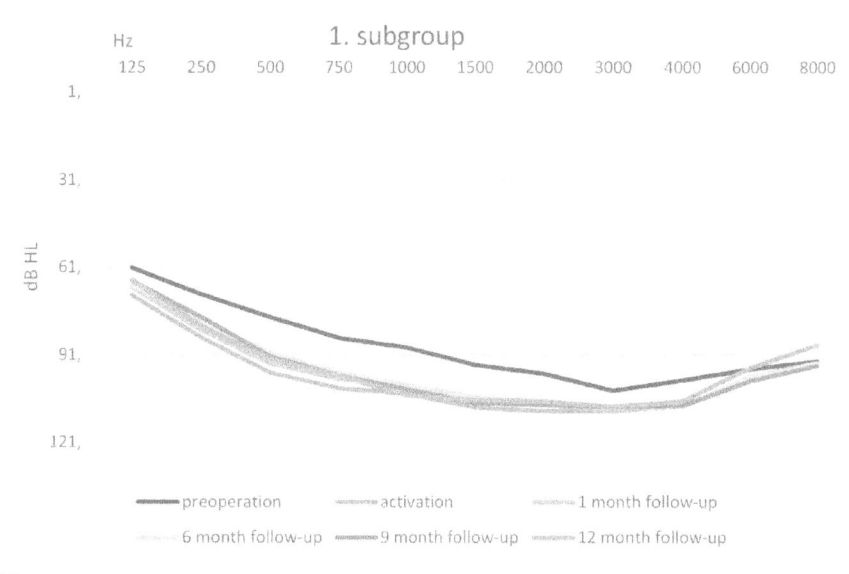

Figure 5.
Average hearing thresholds in patients from the first subgroup with standard steroid treatment in the preoperative period, upon activation, at 1, 6, 9, and 12 months after CI.

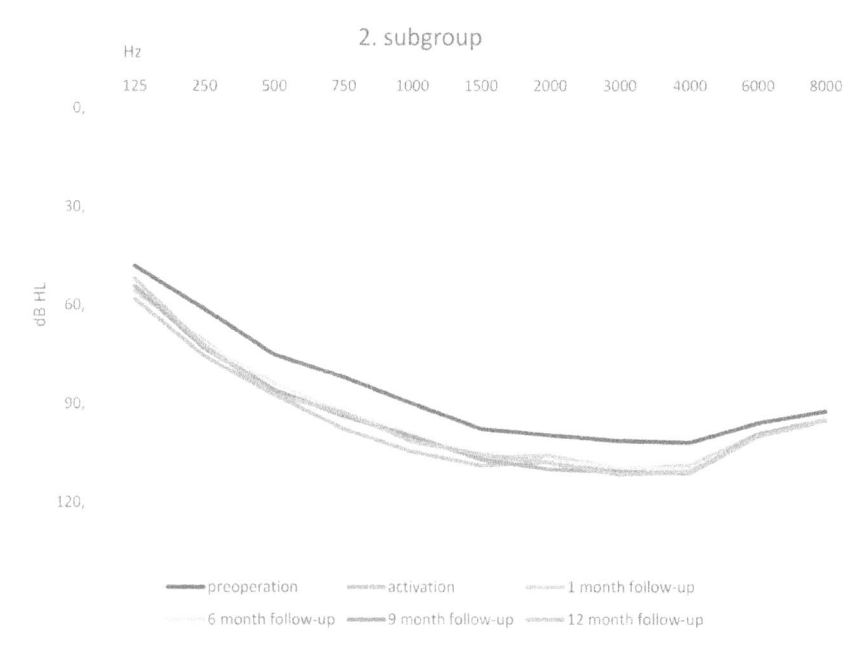

Figure 6.
Average hearing thresholds in patients from the second subgroup with combined steroid treatment in the preoperative period, upon activation, at 1, 6, 9, and 12 months after CI.

of results and the highest overall hearing preservation rate (38%) was observed in the second subgroup. All patients from the second subgroup (prolonged steroid treatment) and almost 69% of patients from the first subgroup had partially or fully preserved hearing. The majority of patients from the control group had minimal HP at 70.6% (see **Table 1** and **Figure 9**).

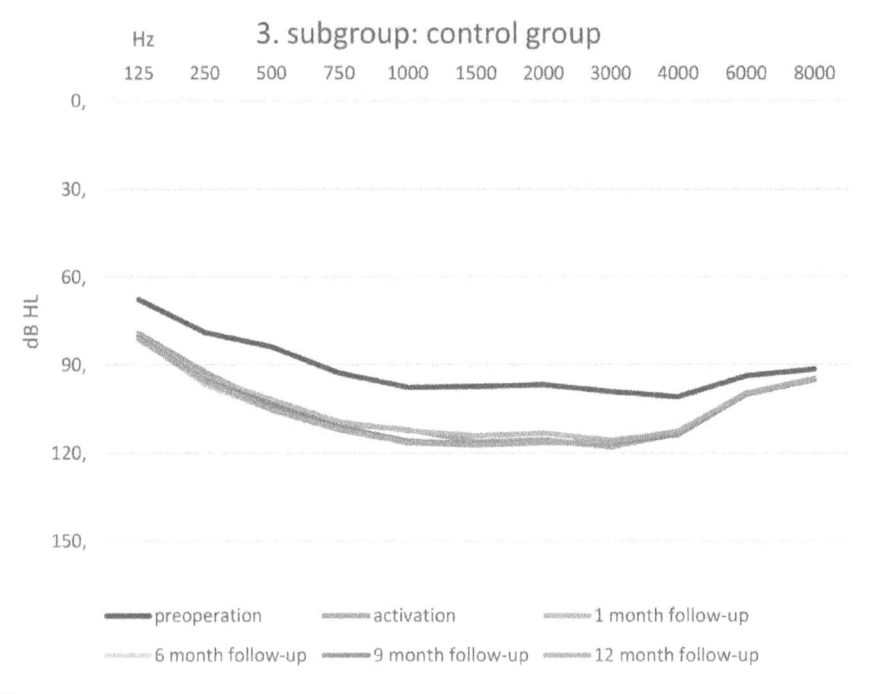

Figure 7.
Average hearing thresholds in patients from the third subgroup (control) with standard steroid treatment in the preoperative period, upon activation, at 1, 6, 9, and 12 months after CI.

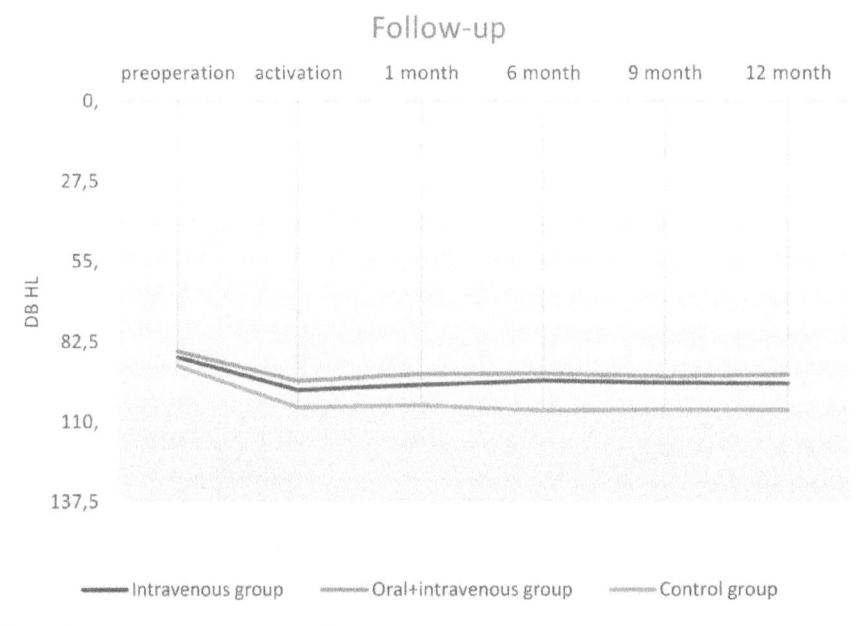

Figure 8.
Average hearing thresholds in patients with standard steroid treatment (group 1), patients with prolonged steroid treatment (group 2), and control (group 3) in the preoperative period, upon activation, at 1, 6, 9, and 12 months after CI.

	Minimal HP (0–25%)	Partial HP (26%–75%)	Complete HP (75%-100%)
Subgroup 1	5 (31.2%)	7 (43.8%)	4 (25.0%)
Subgroup 2	0 (0.0%)	8 (61.5%)	5 (38.5%)
Control Group	12 (70.6%)	3 (17.6%)	2 (11.8%)

Table 1.
HP measured 12 months after implantation, in relation to the therapy applied – the number and percent of patients.

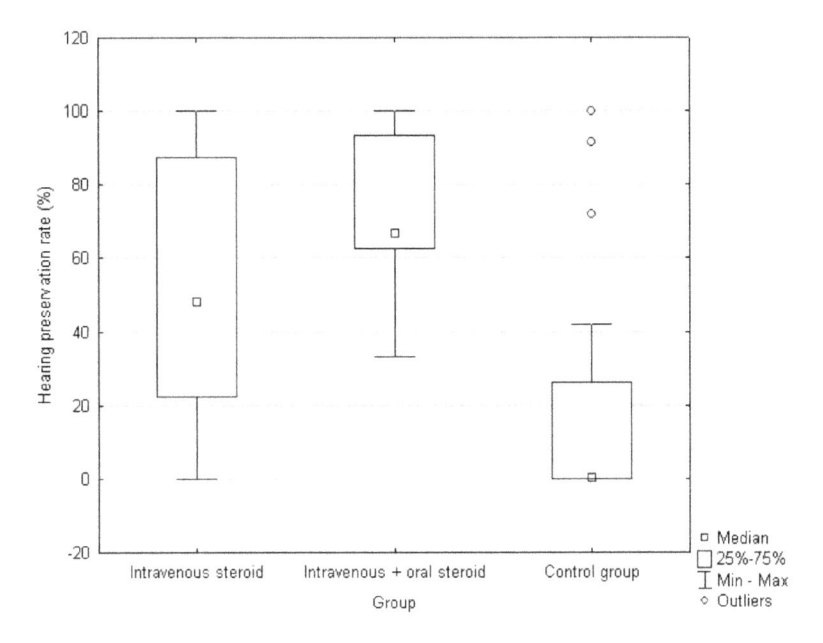

Figure 9.
Hearing preservation rate (HP) in three subgroups.

8. Summary

The role of glicocorticosteroids in the treatment of ENT diseases is very important. According to the results of this study have clearly shown the effect of steroids (dexamethasone and dexamethasone/prednisone) in stabilizing mean hearing thresholds in both experimental subgroups in comparison with the control subgroup during CI. In the preoperative period, the hearing thresholds of participants in all three subgroups were statistically indistinguishable. During the cochlear implantation, the appropriate scheme of pharmacology (corticosteroids) next to the surgical technique and the technology of cochlear implants are key in the cochlear implantation. The corticosteroids play an important role in the pharmacological treatment in different otorhinolaryngological disorders such as Sudden Sensorineural Hearing Loss (SSNHL), Meniere's Disease (MD), Tinnitus and as a supportive treatment in the different ENT (ear-nose-throat) surgery procedures, including cochlear implantation (CI). The effectiveness of therapy of corticosteroids in otorhinolaryngology depends on many different factors. The main are: the duration of the therapy, occurrence or not of adverse reactions, especially in those patients with additional risk factors as comorbidities.

Conflict of interest

The authors declare no conflict of interest.

Abbreviations

MD	Meniere's Disease
SSNHL	Sudden Sensorineural Hearing Loss
ENT	Ear-Nose-Throat
BLB	Blood-Labyrinth-Barrier
CI	Cochlear Implantation
CS	Corticosteroids
LADME	L – liberation; A – absorption; D – distribution; M – metabolism; E – elimination
RWM	Round Window Membrane
DEX	Dexamethasone
QOL	Quality of Life
RCT	Randomized Clinical Trial(s)
PDT	Partial Deafness Treatment
PDT–EC	Partial Deafness Treatment – Electrical Stimulation
PDT–EAS	Partial Deafness Treatment – Electro-Acoustic Stimulation

Author details

Magdalena B. Skarzynska[1,2]* and Piotr H. Skarzynski[1,3,4]

1 Institute of Sensory Organs, Kajetany, Poland

2 Center of Hearing and Speech Medincus, Kajetany, Poland

3 Department of Teleaudiology and Screening, World Hearing Center, Institute of Physiology and Pathology of Hearing, Warsaw, Poland

4 Department of Heart Failure and Cardiac Rehabilitation, Medical University of Warsaw, Poland

*Address all correspondence to: m.skarzynska@medincus.pl

IntechOpen

© 2021 The Author(s). Licensee IntechOpen. This chapter is distributed under the terms of the Creative Commons Attribution License (http://creativecommons.org/licenses/by/3.0), which permits unrestricted use, distribution, and reproduction in any medium, provided the original work is properly cited.

References

[1] Nyberg S, Abbott NJ, Shi X, Steyger PS, Dabdoub A. Delivery of therapeutics to the inner ear: The challenge of the blood-labyrinth barrier. Science Translational Medicine. 2019 Mar 6;11(482):eaao0935.

[2] Salt AN, Plontke SK. Pharmacokinetic principles in the inner ear: Influence of drug properties on intratympanic applications. Hearing Research. 2018 Oct;368:28-40.

[3] Hamid M, Trune D. Issues, indications, and controversies regarding intratympanic steroid perfusion. Current Opinion in Otolaryngology & Head and Neck Surgery. 2008 Oct 1;16(5):434-40.

[4] Liu H, Hao J, Li KS. Current strategies for drug delivery to the inner ear. Acta Pharmaceutica Sinica B. 2013 Apr 1;3(2):86-96.

[5] Clinic of Otorhinolaryngology Alaca State Hospital, Corum, Turkey, Senturk E, Tugrul S, Department of Otorhinolaryngology, Bezmialem Vakif University School of Medicine, Istanbul, Turkey, Yildirim YS, Department of Otorhinolaryngology, Bezmialem Vakif University School of Medicine, Istanbul, Turkey, et al. Are There Any Systemic Effects of the Intratympanic Administration of Dexamethasone? Bezmialem Science. 2018 Sep 21;6(3):186-90.

[6] Rah YC, Lee MY, Kim SH, Kim DH, Eastwood H, O'Leary SJ, et al. Extended use of systemic steroid is beneficial in preserving hearing in guinea pigs after cochlear implant. Acta Otolaryngol. 2016;136(12):1213-9.

[7] Sweeney AD, Carlson ML, Zuniga MG, Bennett ML, Wanna GB, Haynes DS, et al. Impact of Perioperative Oral Steroid Use on Low-frequency Hearing Preservation After Cochlear Implantation. Otol Neurotol. 2015;36(9):1480-5.

[8] O'Leary SJ, Monksfield P, Kel G, Connolly T, Souter MA, Chang A, et al. Relations between cochlear histopathology and hearing loss in experimental cochlear implantation. Hearing Research. 2013 Apr 1;298:27-35.

[9] Hamid M, Trune D. Issues, indications, and controversies regarding intratympanic steroid perfusion. Curr Opin Otolaryngol Head Neck Surg. 2008 Oct;16(5):434-40.

[10] Nyberg S, Abbott NJ, Shi X, Steyger PS, Dabdoub A. Delivery of therapeutics to the inner ear: The challenge of the blood-labyrinth barrier. Sci Transl Med. 2019 Mar 6;11(482).

[11] Salt AN, Plontke SK. Pharmacokinetic principles in the inner ear: Influence of drug properties on intratympanic applications. Hear Res. 2018 Oct;368: 28-40.

[12] Skarżyńska MB, Skarżyński PH, Król B, Kozieł M, Osińska K, Gos E, et al. Preservation of Hearing Following Cochlear Implantation Using Different Steroid Therapy Regimens: A Prospective Clinical Study. Med Sci Monit. 2018 Apr 22;24:2437-45.

[13] Wright T. Menière's disease. BMJ Clin Evid. 2015 Nov 5;2015.

[14] Patel M, Agarwal K, Arshad Q, Hariri M, Rea P, Seemungal BM, et al. Intratympanic methylprednisolone versus gentamicin in patients with unilateral Ménière's disease: a randomised, double-blind, comparative effectiveness trial. Lancet. 2016 Dec 3;388(10061):2753-62.

[15] Dong SH, Kim SS, Kim SH, Yeo SG. Expression of aquaporins in inner ear disease. The Laryngoscope. 2020; 130(6):1532-9.

[16] Espinosa-Sanchez JM, Lopez-Escamez JA. The pharmacological

management of vertigo in Meniere disease. Expert Opin Pharmacother. 2020;21(14):1753-63.

[17] Farhood Z, Lambert PR. The physiologic role of corticosteroids in Ménière's disease. American Journal of Otolaryngology. 2016 Sep 1;37(5):455-8.

[18] Bird PA, Murray DP, Zhang M, Begg EJ. Intratympanic versus intravenous delivery of dexamethasone and dexamethasone sodium phosphate to cochlear perilymph. Otol Neurotol. 2011 Aug;32(6):933-6.

[19] Masoumi E, Dabiri S, Khorsandi Ashtiani MT, Erfanian R, Sohrabpour S, Yazdani N, et al. Methylprednisolone versus Dexamethasone for Control of Vertigo in Patients with Definite Meniere's disease. Iran J Otorhinolaryngol. 2017 Nov;29(95):341-6.

[20] Salt AN, Hartsock JJ, Hou J, Piu F. Comparison of the Pharmacokinetic Properties of Triamcinolone and Dexamethasone for Local Therapy of the Inner Ear. Front Cell Neurosci. 2019; 13:347.

[21] Albu S, Nagy A, Doros C, Marceanu L, Cozma S, Musat G, et al. Treatment of Meniere's disease with intratympanic dexamethazone plus high dosage of betahistine. Am J Otolaryngol. 2016 Jun;37(3):225-30.

[22] Barrs DM. Intratympanic injections of dexamethasone for long-term control of vertigo. Laryngoscope. 2004 Nov; 114(11):1910-4.

[23] Boleas-Aguirre MS, Lin FR, Della Santina CC, Minor LB, Carey JP. Longitudinal results with intratympanic dexamethasone in the treatment of Ménière's disease. Otol Neurotol. 2008 Jan;29(1):33-8.

[24] Casani AP, Piaggi P, Cerchiai N, Seccia V, Franceschini SS, Dallan I. Intratympanic treatment of intractable unilateral Meniere disease: gentamicin or dexamethasone? A randomized controlled trial. Otolaryngol Head Neck Surg. 2012 Mar;146(3):430-7.

[25] Garduño-Anaya MA, Couthino De Toledo H, Hinojosa-González R, Pane-Pianese C, Ríos-Castañeda LC. Dexamethasone inner ear perfusion by intratympanic injection in unilateral Ménière's disease: a two-year prospective, placebo-controlled, double-blind, randomized trial. Otolaryngol Head Neck Surg. 2005 Aug;133(2):285-94.

[26] Herraiz C, Plaza G, Aparicio JM, Gallego I, Marcos S, Ruiz C. Trans-tympanic steroids for Ménière's disease. Otol Neurotol. 2010 Jan;31(1):162-7.

[27] Leng Y, Liu B, Zhou R, Liu J, Liu D, Zhang S-L, et al. Repeated courses of intratympanic dexamethasone injection are effective for intractable Meniere's disease. Acta Otolaryngol. 2017 Feb;137(2):154-60.

[28] Martin Sanz E, Zschaeck C, Christiane ZL, Gonzalez M, Manuel GJ, Mato T, et al. Control of vertigo after intratympanic corticoid therapy for unilateral Ménière's disease: a comparison of weekly versus daily fixed protocols. Otol Neurotol. 2013 Oct;34(8):1429-33.

[29] Martin-Sanz E, Luzardo CZ, Riesco LR, Patino TM, Sanz R. The use of electrocochleography to monitor the response of Ménière's disease patients to intratympanic steroids. Acta Otolaryngol. 2013 Nov;133(11):1158-64.

[30] McRackan TR, Best J, Pearce EC, Bennett ML, Dietrich M, Wanna GB, et al. Intratympanic dexamethasone as a symptomatic treatment for Ménière's disease. Otol Neurotol. 2014 Oct;35(9): 1638-40.

[31] She W, Lv L, Du X, Li H, Dai Y, Lu L, et al. Long-term effects of intratympanic methylprednisolone perfusion treatment on intractable

[32] Lambert PR, Nguyen S, Maxwell KS, Tucci DL, Lustig LR, Fletcher M, et al. A randomized, double-blind, placebo-controlled clinical study to assess safety and clinical activity of OTO-104 given as a single intratympanic injection in patients with unilateral Ménière's disease. Otol Neurotol. 2012 Sep;33(7):1257-65.

[33] Lambert PR, Carey J, Mikulec AA, LeBel C. Intratympanic Sustained-Exposure Dexamethasone Thermo-sensitive Gel for Symptoms of Ménière's Disease: Randomized Phase 2b Safety and Efficacy Trial. Otol Neurotol. 2016 Dec;37(10):1669-76.

[34] Devantier L, Djurhuus BD, Hougaard DD, Händel MN, Guldfred FL-A, Schmidt JH, et al. Intratympanic Steroid for Ménière's Disease: A Systematic Review. Otol Neurotol. 2019 Jul;40(6):806-12.

[35] Frejo L, Martin-Sanz E, Teggi R, Trinidad G, Soto-Varela A, Santos-Perez S, et al. Extended phenotype and clinical subgroups in unilateral Meniere disease: A cross-sectional study with cluster analysis. Clin Otolaryngol. 2017 Dec;42(6):1172-80.

[36] Frejo L, Soto-Varela A, Santos-Perez S, Aran I, Batuecas-Caletrio A, Perez-Guillen V, et al. Clinical Subgroups in Bilateral Meniere Disease. Front Neurol. 2016;7:182.

[37] Leung MA, Flaherty A, Zhang JA, Hara J, Barber W, Burgess L. Sudden Sensorineural Hearing Loss: Primary Care Update. Hawaii J Med Public Health. 2016 Jun;75(6):172-4.

[38] Wei BP, Stathopoulos D, O'Leary S. Steroids for idiopathic sudden sensorineural hearing loss. Cochrane Database Syst Rev [Internet]. 2013 Jul 2 [cited 2021 Mar 29];2013(7). Available from: https://www.ncbi.nlm.nih.gov/pmc/articles/PMC7390468/

[39] Chandrasekhar SS, Tsai Do BS, Schwartz SR, Bontempo LJ, Faucett EA, Finestone SA, et al. Clinical Practice Guideline: Sudden Hearing Loss (Update). Otolaryngol Head Neck Surg. 2019 Aug;161(1_suppl):S1-45.

[40] Ermutlu G, Süslü N, Yılmaz T, Saraç S. Sudden hearing loss: an effectivity comparison of intratympanic and systemic steroid treatments. Eur Arch Otorhinolaryngol. 2017 Oct 1;274(10):3585-91.

[41] Hong SM, Park CH, Lee JH. Hearing outcomes of daily intratympanic dexamethasone alone as a primary treatment modality for ISSHL. Otolaryngol Head Neck Surg. 2009 Nov;141(5):579-83.

[42] Lim HJ, Kim YT, Choi SJ, Lee JB, Park HY, Park K, et al. Efficacy of 3 different steroid treatments for sudden sensorineural hearing loss: a prospective, randomized trial. Otolaryngol Head Neck Surg. 2013 Jan;148(1):121-7.

[43] Mirian C, Ovesen T. Intratympanic vs Systemic Corticosteroids in First-line Treatment of Idiopathic Sudden Sensorineural Hearing Loss. JAMA Otolaryngol Head Neck Surg. 2020 May;146(5):1-8.

[44] Rauch SD, Halpin CF, Antonelli PJ, Babu S, Carey JP, Gantz BJ, et al. Oral vs intratympanic corticosteroid therapy for idiopathic sudden sensorineural hearing loss: a randomized trial. JAMA. 2011 May 25;305(20):2071-9.

[45] Swachia K, Sharma D, Singh J. Efficacy of oral vs. intratympanic corticosteroids in sudden sensorineural hearing loss. J Basic Clin Physiol Pharmacol. 2016 Jun 1;27(4):371-7.

[46] Tsounis M, Psillas G, Tsalighopoulos M, Vital V, Maroudias N,

Markou K. Systemic, intratympanic and combined administration of steroids for sudden hearing loss. A prospective randomized multicenter trial. Eur Arch Otorhinolaryngol. 2018 Jan;275(1): 103-10.

[47] Battaglia A, Burchette R, Cueva R. Combination therapy (intratympanic dexamethasone + high-dose prednisone taper) for the treatment of idiopathic sudden sensorineural hearing loss. Otol Neurotol. 2008 Jun;29(4):453-60.

[48] Crane RA, Camilon M, Nguyen S, Meyer TA. Steroids for treatment of sudden sensorineural hearing loss: a meta-analysis of randomized controlled trials. Laryngoscope. 2015 Jan;125(1): 209-17.

[49] Dahm V, Nieratschker M, Riss D, Kaider A, Auinger A, Honeder C, et al. Intratympanic Triamcinolone Acetonide as Treatment Option for Idiopathic Sudden Sensorineural Hearing Loss. Otol Neurotol. 2019 Jul;40(6):720-7.

[50] Alexander TH, Harris JP, Nguyen QT, Vorasubin N. Dose Effect of Intra-tympanic Dexamethasone for Idiopathic Sudden Sensorineural Hearing Loss: 24 mg/mL Is Superior to 10 mg/mL. Otol Neurotol. 2015 Sep;36(8):1321-7.

[51] Tunkel DE, Bauer CA, Sun GH, Rosenfeld RM, Chandrasekhar SS, Cunningham ER, et al. Clinical Practice Guideline: Tinnitus. Otolaryngol Head Neck Surg. 2014 Oct 1;151(2_suppl): S1-40.

[52] Yener HM, Sarı E, Aslan M, Yollu U, Gözen ED, İnci E. The Efficacy of Intratympanic Steroid Injection in Tinnitus Cases Unresponsive to Medical Treatment. J Int Adv Otol. 2020 Aug; 16(2):197-200.

[53] Araújo MFS, Oliveira CA, Bahmad FM. Intratympanic dexamethasone injections as a treatment for severe, disabling tinnitus: does it work? Arch Otolaryngol Head Neck Surg. 2005 Feb;131(2):113-7.

[54] Choi SJ, Lee JB, Lim HJ, In SM, Kim J-Y, Bae KH, et al. Intratympanic dexamethasone injection for refractory tinnitus: prospective placebo-controlled study. Laryngoscope. 2013 Nov;123(11): 2817-22.

[55] She W, Dai Y, Du X, Chen F, Ding X, Cui X. Treatment of subjective tinnitus: a comparative clinical study of intra-tympanic steroid injection vs. oral carbamazepine. Med Sci Monit. 2009 Jun;15(6):PI35-39.

[56] Topak M, Sahin-Yilmaz A, Ozdoganoglu T, Yilmaz HB, Ozbay M, Kulekci M. Intratympanic methyl-prednisolone injections for subjective tinnitus. J Laryngol Otol. 2009 Nov;123(11):1221-5.

[57] Shim HJ, Song SJ, Choi AY, Hyung Lee R, Yoon SW. Comparison of various treatment modalities for acute tinnitus. Laryngoscope. 2011 Dec;121(12): 2619-25.

[58] Albu S, Chirtes F. Intratympanic dexamethasone plus melatonin versus melatonin only in the treatment of unilateral acute idiopathic tinnitus. Am J Otolaryngol. 2014 Oct;35(5):617-22.

[59] Lee H-J, Kim M-B, Yoo S-Y, Park SN, Nam E-C, Moon IS, et al. Clinical effect of intratympanic dexamethasone injection in acute unilateral tinnitus: A prospective, placebo-controlled, multicenter study. Laryngoscope. 2018 Jan;128(1):184-8.

[60] Diao M, Sun J, Tian F, Xu S, Jia Z, Liu Y, et al. [Effect of postaurical subcutaneously injection of triamcinolone acetonide for subjective tinnitus]. Zhonghua Yi Xue Za Zhi. 2013 Nov 12;93(42):3384-7.

[61] Skarzynski H, van de Heyning P, Agrawal S, Arauz SL, Atlas M,

Baumgartner W, et al. Towards a consensus on a hearing preservation classification system. Acta Otolaryngol Suppl. 2013;(564):3-13.

[62] Skarżyńska MB, Skarżyński PH, Król B, Kozieł M, Osińska K, Gos E, et al. Preservation of Hearing Following Cochlear Implantation Using Different Steroid Therapy Regimens: A Prospective Clinical Study. Medical Science Monitor : International Medical Journal of Experimental and Clinical Research. 2018;24:2437.

[63] Skarżyński H, Lorens A, Skarżyński PH. Electro-Natural Stimulation (ENS) in Partial Deafness Treatment: A case study. JHS. 2014;4(4): 67-71.

Chapter 4

Pharmacogenomics and Pharmacotranscriptomics of Glucocorticoids in Pediatric Acute Lymphoblastic Leukemia

Vladimir Gasic, Djordje Pavlovic, Biljana Stankovic, Nikola Kotur, Branka Zukic and Sonja Pavlovic

Abstract

Pharmacogenomics and pharmacotranscriptomics contribute to more efficient and safer treatment of many diseases, especially malignancies. Acute lymphoblastic leukemia (ALL) is the most common hematological malignancy during childhood. Glucocorticoids, prednisone and dexamethasone, represent the basis of chemotherapy in pediatric ALL. Therapy causes side effects in 75% of patients and 1–3% of pediatric ALL patients die because of therapy side effects rather than the disease itself. Due to this fact, pharmacogenomics and pharmacotranscriptomics have gained key positions in this field. There is a growing knowledge of pharmacogenomics and pharmacotranscriptomics markers relevant for the success of the glucocorticoid treatment of children with ALL. New technologies, such as next-generation sequencing (NGS) have created a possibility for designing panels of pharmacogenomics and pharmacotranscriptomics markers related to the response to glucocorticoid drugs. Optimization of these panels through population pharmacogenomic studies leads to new knowledge that could open the doors widely to pre-emptive pharmacogenomic testing.

Keywords: glucocorticoids, pediatric acute lymphoblastic leukemia, pharmacogenomics, pharmacotranscriptomics, population pharmacogenomics

1. Introduction

Personalized medicine has always been applied in good medical practice. Nowadays, with the development of medicine and molecular biology, personalized medicine, also known as precision medicine, has become an integral component of modern medicine. Fascinating methodological advancements, especially an improvement of high throughput "omics" analysis, has led to the conclusion that genomic and transcriptomic profiling can bring about not only knowledge concerning the causes of multiple diseases that aren't traumas or infections, but also information that could contribute to the specificities of treatment of each individual. Thus, personalized medicine is aiming to provide the most efficient and the least harmful (toxic) treatment protocol to each patient [1, 2].

Among the subfields which could contribute to the formation of these individual protocols are the subfields of pharmacogenomics and pharmacotranscriptomics.

Pharmacogenomics deals with research whose results need to show if there are any associations between the variations in the genome and the efficacy or toxicity of a certain drug. Pharmacotranscriptomics deals with research that needs to determine if there are associations between the variations in the transcriptome and the efficacy or toxicity of a drug.

Specific genes and transcripts related to metabolizing enzyme gene variants, drug transporter gene variants, and gene variants that have been related to a predisposition to certain adverse events, might influence the response of a patient to a drug.

According to the U.S. Food and Drug Administration (FDA), there are many patients who would benefit if a health care provider considered pharmacogenomic testing before prescribing an appropriate drug or drug dosage. Up to date there are more than 50 drugs for which the gene-drug interaction data support therapeutic management recommendations, and more than 30 drugs for which the gene-drug interaction data indicate a potential impact on safety or response [3].

Aside from that, pharmacogenomics and pharmacotranscriptomics also try to identify markers associated with a disease, which can be targets for new therapeutics (molecularly-targeted therapy, gene-therapy).

The ultimate goal of pharmacogenomics and pharmacotranscriptomics is to create optimal therapy strategy based on the genomic and transcriptomic profile of a patient.

2. Pharmacogenomics and pharmacotranscriptomics of glucocorticoids in pediatric acute lymphoblastic leukemia

2.1 Pediatric acute lymphoblastic leukemia

Pediatric acute lymphoblastic leukemia (ALL), a pathological increased proliferation of lymphoid progenitors, lymphoblasts, is the most common neoplasm among children and it is also the one with the highest rate of complete remission, which covers up to 85% of the patients treated with modern protocols [4, 5].

Unfortunately, unwanted treatment effects occur in about 75% of patients [6]. Studies estimate that about 1–2% of pediatric ALL patients have a lethal outcome due to treatment [7].

There are several treatment protocols for pediatric ALL, consisting of the similar phases: remission induction and early intensification, consolidation, reinduction and maintenance. Standard treatment protocols for pediatric ALL include several commonly used drugs, i.e. glucocorticoids, vincristine, asparaginase, anthracyclines, thiopurines and methotrexate [5, 8, 9].

2.2 Glucocorticoid treatment of pediatric acute lymphoblastic leukemia

Synthetics glucocorticoids (GCs) are capable of inducing apoptosis in thymocytes, monocytes, and peripheral T cells. GC drugs, prednisone and dexamethasone, represent the basis of chemotherapy in pediatric ALL because of their cytotoxic and antiproliferative effect.

According to the Berlin-Frankfurt-Munster protocol, the pediatric ALL protocol specific for Europe, GCs are used in the remission induction phase of treatment. The primary goal of this phase is to use GCs to promote apoptosis in order to significantly lower the number of lymphoblasts. The number of blasts in the peripheral blood on the 8th day is an important prognostic marker. Also, GCs are used after the consolidation phase, if a marrow relapse during or shortly following initial continuation chemotherapy is developed. GCs are administered in the first phase of reinduction (day 1–36), in order to achieve a second complete remission [10].

Inter-individual differences in the efficiency and adverse effects of GCs in children with ALL have been observed. A study on dexamethasone pharmacokinetics following treatment of children with ALL showed large inter-patient variability, with a greater than ten-fold variability in systemic drug exposure observed at a dose of 8 mg/m2/d [11]. Also, there are still 57% of patients who have poor response to prednisone, and resistance to prednisone has become one of the main obstacles to achieve successful treatment outcomes in pediatric ALL [7].

It is for this reason that pharmacogenomics and pharmacotranscriptomics became very important in GC treatment of pediatric ALL patients [12].

2.3 Pharmacogenomics markers

2.3.1 NR3C1 gene

The first pharmacogene to be studied in relation to GC sensitivity is the *NR3C1* gene that encodes the glucocorticoid receptor (GR). Four variants in this gene have been associated with variation in sensitivity to GCs, two of which contribute to a decrease in sensitivity, while the other two contribute to an increase in sensitivity [13]. Although initially these variants were shown to have no association with differences in response to GC therapy in childhood ALL, later studies with a greater number of study subjects have had different findings [14].

The variant rs56149945 (N363S) is an A > G missense variant in exon 2, which causes an asparagine to serine amino acid substitution in position 363 in the N-terminal domain of the receptor. The minor allele of this variant has been associated with increased sensitivity to GCs, resulting in increased body mass index and lower bone mineral density [15]. A proposed mechanism for this sensitivity is that the new serine residue becomes a target of phosphorylation, changing the phosphorylation state of the receptor [16]. Microarray analysis revealed a unique, variant-specific pattern of gene regulation for N363S when compared to wild-type GR [17]. In a study on childhood ALL, N363S carriers were found to be more prone to steroid-related toxicity during GC therapy, however they were also better prednisone responders overall, and had better 5-year event-free survival rates, supporting the idea that this variant causes increased sensitivity [18].

The variant rs41423247 is also associated with increased sensitivity to dexamethasone. It is a C > G single nucleotide variant in intron 2 that was discovered as a *Bcl*I restriction fragment length polymorphism [19]. It was found that the minor allele of the *Bcl*I variant was associated with good prednisone response in pediatric ALL patients [20]. Along with the *Bcl*I variant, two other variants in intron 2, rs33388 and rs33389, form a three-point ACT haplotype that is associated with increased sensitivity to GCs [21].

The linked variants rs6189/rs6190 (ER22/E23EK) have been associated with resistance to GCs as well as lower insulin, cholesterol and CRP levels [22]. Both variants are G > A single nucleotide substitutions, however variant rs62189 is silent, whereas rs6190 is a missense variant that results in an amino acid change from arginine to lysine. The variants promote expression of the GR-A isoform of GR, which is less transcriptionally active than the GR-B isoform [23]. No significant association of this variant with the therapeutic response to GCs has been found in childhood ALL [14].

Another variant associated with decreased sensitivity is rs6198. It is a A > G single nucleotide variant in exon 9β. The variant is inside an ATTTA motif and promotes alternative splicing resulting in the expression of GRβ. This contributes to decreased sensitivity to GCs since GRβ does not bind GCs and is transcriptionally inactive [24]. It has been shown that the presence of the minor allele of variant rs6198 is associated with poor response to GCs in the initial phase of remission induction therapy in childhood ALL [25].

2.3.2 ABCB1 gene

The *ABCB1* gene (previously known as *MDR1* gene) encodes a membrane transporter P-glycoprotein (PGP), which is an efflux transporter that actively pumps xenobiotics, including GCs, out of the cell. It has been shown that heightened expression of PGP can lead to resistance to GCs, making this an important pharmacogene [26].

A C > T silent variant in exon 26, rs1045642 (also called 3435C > T), has been associated with lower expression and activity of PGP *in vivo*. This leads to higher plasma levels of xenobiotics being retained [27]. The proposed mechanism of lowered expression and activity is that the minor T allele causes mRNA instability, as well as that the presence of a rare codon that it creates, affects cotranslational folding of PGP [28, 29]. The 3435CC genotype has been associated with significantly lower event-free survival and overall survival in ALL patients, showing that the presence of 3435C > T variant is associated with better treatment outcome [30].

Two other variants are in linkage disequilibrium with 3435C > T, rs1128503 (1236C > T) and rs2032582 (2677G > T/A), but it has been shown that they do not account for the change in expression, and have not shown an association with risk of relapse in ALL [31]. However, a rare CGT haplotype (rs1128503-rs2032582-rs1045642) has been associated with high blast count in the initial phase of remission induction therapy [25].

2.3.3 Glutathione S-transferase (GST) genes

Three genes, *GSTM1, GSTT1* and *GSTP1*, encode detoxification enzymes from the glutathione S-transferase family. They catalyze the conjugation of reduced glutathione and xenobiotics, which is the first step in elimination of GCs. This makes GSTs a possible pharmacogenomic marker when it comes to GCs [32].

The main *GSTM1* and *GSTT1* genotype variants are inherited homozygous deletions of the gene (null genotype), resulting in an absence of enzyme activity. The evidence on how they affect therapy outcome in ALL is conflicting. The earliest study found that *GSTT1* null, but not *GSTM1* null genotype was associated with a reduction in risk of poor response to prednisone [33]. It was also shown that the simultaneous deletion of both the *GSTM1* and *GSTT1* genes was found to be more predictive than any other parameter of early relapse of childhood B-precursor ALL [34]. A later study showed the *GSTM1* null genotype was associated with better clinical outcome within prednisone poor-responder patients, whereas the *GSTT1* null genotype was associated with worse outcome in the standard-risk group and within prednisone good responders. These findings suggest that the *GSTM1* null genotype has a protective role while the *GSTT1* null genotype has an unfavorable effect in specific subsets of ALL patients [35]. However, the largest study on 710 children with ALL, found no association between *GSTT1* and *GSTM1* null genotypes and treatment outcome [36].

GSTP1 has two most commonly studied variants - rs1695 and rs1138272. Variant rs1695 is a A > G missense variant that causes an isoleucine to valine substitution in position 105 that affects the thermal stability of the enzyme [37]. Variant rs1138272 is a nearby C > T missense variant that causes an alanine to valine substitution in position 114. It has been shown that the GC (rs1695-rs1138272) haplotype was associated with a good response to GCs in the remission induction phase of childhood ALL [25].

2.3.4 Discovery of novel variants

Though the above-mentioned variants account for some variability in response to GC therapy, the research on GC pharmacogenomics is limited, and studies on larger cohorts and accounting for different ALL subgroups are needed. Novel pharmacogene variants could be essential for personalization of GC dose that results in minimal toxicity and maximum cancer cell death [38]. Recently, genome-wide association studies (GWAS) have attempted to discover new variants with potential impact on pharmacogenomics variation of treatment outcome.

One of the adverse effects of GCs is hypertension. A study analyzing 203 candidate polymorphisms aimed to define the genetic risk factors for steroid-induced hypertension. The strongest association was identified with the contactin-associated protein-like-2, *CNTNAP2* (7q35-q36), a gene whose impaired function has been associated with blood pressure, though the mechanism of this association is unclear. Another association with hypertension was with the missense variant rs1137101 (LEPR Gln223Arg). It is found in the *LEPR* gene, that encodes the leptin receptor, whose ligand, leptin, regulates adipose tissue mass and body weight. Three SNPs in the *CRHR1* gene were associated with hypertension. This gene encodes the corticotropin-releasing hormone receptor that mediates the release of the adrenocorticotropic hormone. Carriers of the major rs1876828 G and rs1876829 A alleles and of the minor rs242941 T allele all had a higher incidence of hypertension [39].

Another important adverse effect of GC administration is osteonecrosis. A GWAS study of SNPs in a cohort comprising 2285 children with ALL, found that the presence of minor allele at SNP rs10989692, near the glutamate receptor *GRIN3A* locus, was associated with osteonecrosis. The second highest osteonecrosis-associated ranked variant was in a similar gene, *GRIK1*. These findings point to the involvement of the glutamate pathway in the pathogenesis of GC-induced osteonecrosis [40].

In a GWAS study, 440 044 SNPs were scanned on whether they contributed to the risk of relapse in 2535 childhood ALL patients. Dexamethasone plasma clearance was associated with 4 out of 134 SNPs associated with relapse, 2 of which were within the above mentioned *ABCB1I gene,* and both associated with higher dexamethasone clearance and a higher relapse risk [41].

The Cortisol Network (CORNET) consortium undertook a GWAS meta-analysis for plasma cortisol in 12,597 Caucasian participants, and found that individual differences in morning plasma cortisol levels amongst Europeans can be attributed to genetic variation within a region on chromosome 14. This locus includes *SERPINA6*, which encodes the corticosteroid binding globulin (CBG), the major cortisol-binding protein in plasma, as well as *SERPINA1*, which encodes α1-antitrypsin, a protein that inhibits cleavage of the reactive center loop that releases cortisol from CBG. Three SNPs were identified, some of which were associated with total CBG concentration, while the top hit, rs12589136, was found to influence the immunoreactivity of the reactive center loop of CBG [42]. Research like this gives insight into possible new candidate-gene targets that could be included in an expanding pharmacogenomics panel.

2.4 Pharmacotranscriptomics markers

Aside from the above-mentioned variants that directly affect expression levels, research in the field of pharmacotranscriptomics markers of GC response is still new and insufficient. Recently, the expression level of certain RNAs has been associated with drug response, trying to establish the measuring of RNA expression as a marker of drug response that could guide therapy individualization [12]. A new area of focus is non-coding RNAs (ncRNAs) - transcripts which are not translated into proteins, but whose expression profile is widely altered in many malignancies. Two types of ncRNAs have been studied in relation to GC resistance, long non-coding RNAs (lncRNAs), which are non-coding transcripts longer than 200 nucleotides, and micro-RNAs (miRNAs), which are short transcripts with an important role as post-transcriptional regulators [43].

One lncRNA, GAS5, has been shown to be associated with a poor GC response in childhood ALL during the phase of remission induction therapy [44]. GAS5 is a regulatory tumor-suppressor lncRNA whose expression was first detected in growth-arrested cells. One of the mechanisms by which GAS5 achieves its role is molecular mimicry of the glucocorticoid response element (GRE). This causes GAS5 to compete with the genomic GREs for binding of the GC-GR complex [45]. ALL patients whose number of blasts on day 8 after the start of treatment was below 100 per µL of peripheral blood had a higher GAS5 expression at diagnosis, and those who had a higher ratio of GAS5 expression on day 15 versus after the start of treatment had a higher number of blasts on day 8. This suggests that the expression level of GAS5 could be a potential marker of therapy response in remission induction therapy [44].

One study that used a computational approach based upon emerging biomedical and biological ontologies and semantic technologies was used to investigate the roles of miRNA regulation on GC resistance in childhood ALL. It was found that hsa-miR-142-3p and hsa-miR-17-5p are the two most promising miRNAs related to GC resistance in pediatric ALL [46]. In another study, it was reported that T-cell ALL patients with high expression of hsa-miR-142-3p had a shorter survival time than those with low expression. This was explained by the oncogenic role of hsa-miR-142-3p that was mediated by inducing resistance to GC treatment through targeting GC receptor-α [47]. Down-regulated hsa-miR-17-5p was related to apoptosis induced by dexamethasone in primary *ex vivo* ALL cells. Therefore, hsa-miR-17-5p might play a role in GC-induced cell death and GC resistance in B-cell ALL [48].

2.5 Panel of pharmacogenes and pharmacogenomic variants of glucocorticoid response

In order to design a panel of pharmacogenes and pharmacogenomics variants related to GC therapy, several approaches have been used to identify pharmacogenes and pharmacogenomics markers whose pharmacogenomics potential could be relevant for application in clinical practice [49].

Using the database PharmGKB (www.pharmgkb.org) and searching the literature on the PubMed database, 22 pharmacogenes have been selected in order to create a panel of genes for which there is evidence of their influence on the effects of GCs (**Table 1**).

Further searching of databases and literature has resulted in selecting 18 pharmacovariants for which there is evidence of influence on the effects of GCs (**Table 2**).

Three criteria were applied to evaluate the potential of variants to be pharmacogenomics markers of GCs. First, the classification was performed by the level of evidence according to PharmGKB. Then, only variants with high minor allele frequencies (MAF) were considered, and finally, the third criterion was the assessment of the functional effect of the variant using *in silico* prediction algorithms that estimate the potential influence of an amino acid substitution on the functioning of the proteins which they encode [49].

Assignment of a level of evidence by the PharmGKB annotation scoring system for clinical and variant annotations enables easier identification of significant

ABCB1	FCER2	HSPA4
ADRB2	FKBP5	NCOA3
CREBBP	GSTM1	NR3C1
CRHR1	GSTP1	SERPINA6
CYP3A4	GSTT1	ST13
CYP3A5	HSD11B2	STIP1
CYP3A7	HSP90AA1	TBP
		TBX21

Table 1.
List of pharmacogenes related to GC therapy.

pharmacovariants. The clinical annotation score represents the sum of the scores of all attached variant, guidelines and drug label annotations. Variant annotations are scored depending on: phenotype category, p-value, cohort size, effect size and weighting by study type or by association and significance. Clinical annotation scores do not rank or compare clinical annotations within a given level of evidence. Level 1A clinical annotations designate variant-drug combinations with variant-specific prescribing guidance in a current clinical guideline or an FDA-approved drug label annotation, while level 1B supports the association but without variant-specific prescribing guidance in an annotated clinical guideline or FDA drug label. Variants level 2A belong to known pharmacogenes, listed in PharmGKB's Very Important Pharmacogenes (VIPs), and describe variant-drug combinations with a substantial evidence to support their importance. Variants level 2B clinical annotations describe variant-drug combinations with a moderate level of evidence supporting the association and not listed in PharmGKB's VIPs. Level 3 clinical annotations describe variant-drug combinations based on a single study or on preliminary results. In level 4 clinical annotations, variant-drug combinations total score is negative with no evidence to support an association between the variant and the drug phenotype [50].

For the evaluation of the pharmacogenomic potential of the selected variants, the level of evidence that correspond to association of each variant to drug response is extracted from PharmGKB database. Evidence level 1 corresponds to highest degree of certainty, while higher numbers correspond to lower degree of evidence for a variant-drug pair. Only variants with MAF higher than 10% have been considered as good candidates for pharmacovariants. Also, only exon variants, whose pharmacogenomics potential in GC therapy has already been confirmed in earlier studies, have been considered.

However, none of the selected variants have enough evidence to support the claim that they have sufficient pharmacogenomics potential in order to be included in the protocols of treatment where GCs are used. The PharmGKB level of evidence was 3 for several variants, but most of them had only variant annotation scores. Even among variants that are in exons, only a few have been predicted to impact the structure and/or function of encoded proteins (probably damaging). Some of the variants have a high MAF. However, none of them completely fulfilled the criteria for a pharmacogenomics variant. Therefore, there is no basis to include any of these variants in clinical practice.

To conclude, up to now, there is not enough indication for any pharmacogenomics marker to be recommended for pre-emptive genetic testing when GCs are administered, and they cannot be introduced in clinical practice.

The transcriptome consists of various coding mRNAs and non-coding RNAs. The content of the transcriptome is inconsistent. It depends on alternative splicing, RNA editing and alternative transcription. It can vary with environmental conditions and the time point of transcriptome profiling has to be considered for the establishment of the transcriptome data. Therefore, the introduction of

rs number[1]	Gene	Variant	PharmGKB[2]	MAF[3]	Effect[4]
rs2229109	ABCB1	c.1199G > A (p.Ser400Asn)	Level 3	3.3%	Benign
rs1128503	ABCB1	c.1236 T > C (p.Gly412=)	VA	41.6%	NA
rs2032582	ABCB1	c.2677G > T/A (p.Ser893Ala/Thr)	Level 3	42.7%	Benign
rs1045642	ABCB1	c.3435 T > C/A (p.Ile1145Met/Ile)	Level 3	51.8%	Prob.* Damag.
rs1042713	ADRB2	c.46G > A (p.Gly16Arg)	Level 3	38.6%	Benign
rs1695	GSTP1	c.313A > G (p.Ile105Val)	VA	66.9%	Benign
rs1138272	GSTP1	c.341C > T (p.Ala114Val)	VA	7.1%	Benign
rs10873531	HSP90AA1	c.282 C > T (p.Thr94=)	VA	88.1%	NA
rs6195	NR3C1	c.1088A > G (p.Asn363Ser)	VA	1.8%	Benign
rs104893913	NR3C1	c.1433G > A (p.Arg478His)	VA	0.00039%	Prob. Damag.
rs6194	NR3C1	c.1767C > T (p.His589=)	VA	0.2%	NA
rs138896520	NR3C1	c.1899G > A (p.Gln633=)	VA	0.0014%	NA
rs72558023	NR3C1	c.198A > G (p.Pro66=)	VA	0.00079%	NA
rs6196	NR3C1	c.2301 T > C (p.Asn767=)	VA	14.9%	NA
rs6189	NR3C1	c.66G > A (p.Glu22Asp)	VA	3%	Benign
rs72542742	NR3C1	c.685G > A (p.Ala229Thr)	VA	0.1%	Benign
rs6190	NR3C1	c.68G > A (p.Arg23Lys)	VA	3%	Benign
rs2240017	TBX21	c.99C > G (p.His33Gln)	Level 3	2%	Benign

[1]rs number: a reference SNP ID number of SNPs that map to an identical location assigned by NCBI.
[2]PharmGKB Level of Evidence: score of pharmacogenomics variant relevance that includes both clinical and variant annotation scores. Level 1: the highest, level 4: the lowest variant-drug evidence association. VA: variant annotation.
[3]MAF: minor allele frequency.
[4]Effect is estimated using PolyPhen-2; a tool for prediction of possible impact of an amino acid substitution on the structure and function of a human protein based on a number of features comprising the sequence, phylogenetic and structural information characterizing the substitution.
*Refers to minor allele C; NA – non applicable.

Table 2.
Pharmacovariants related to GC therapy.

pharmacotranscriptomics markers in the panel possibly used for pre-emptive testing, in order to optimize GC use at the point of prescribing, will be very challenging.

2.6 Population pharmacogenomics

The more investigations were performed in the field of pharmacogenomics, the more prominent became the differences between different ethnical groups when it came to drug response. Due to this fact, it was no longer possible to use data gained from investigating one population in order to apply it to another population [51]. A good example of variability between populations, which has pharmacogenomics significance is the deficiency of the enzyme glucose-6-phosphate-dehydrogenase (G6PD), responsible for the response to unwanted, toxic effects of the drug primaquine. There is a significantly higher number of G6PD-deficient carriers in the population the dark-skinned people of Africa, compared to the white skinned population of America. The prevalence of this genetic marker in Africa is a result of selective pressure, since the carriers of this variant cannot contract malaria, a common cause of death on this continent [52].

Individualization of therapy, as a practical application of knowledge from pharmacogenomics, has been based on studies performed on the populations of white skinned people. When other ethnical groups were included in the clinical investigations, the data led to the conclusion that an individual's ethnic background can influence the response of the individual to different therapeutics. Since the metabolism of drugs is population-specific, data gained from studies performed on one population cannot be extrapolated on the rest. Understanding the pharmacogenomics differences between populations can be of great importance for the pharmaceutical industry and for reducing costs of treatment and overall performances of health systems of any country [53].

Population pharmacogenomics studies enable the integration of pharmacogenomics into health care systems around the world and give a strong support to pre-emptive pharmacogenomics testing [54]. Transcriptome variation in the human population has rarely been studied and there is no evidence on the studies of its application in pharmacotrascriptomics.

2.7 Discovery of new potential pharmacogenomic markers of glucocorticoid response

Novel high-throughput methodology for genomic profiling, especially next-generation sequencing (NGS), has provided a great amount of data that can be a source for bioinformatics analysis. New knowledge can be gained using these modern approaches. They can also be used for the discovery of new potential pharmacogenomics markers.

Analysis of known pharmacogenes related to GC therapy for potential novel pharmacogenomics markers can be performed using two criteria: a prediction algorithm (such as Polyphen-2) showing that the variant affects the protein function, and the frequency of the altered (minor) allele being high.

Population pharmacogenomics study can be helpful in this effort because if the MAF is considerably high in a certain population for some potential new pharmacogenomics marker, validation and clinical studies are strongly encouraged.

One of the most comprehensive human genome database, "1000 genomes" has been searched, and two variants in known pharmacogenes related to GC therapy that could be interesting for validation studies and clinical association studies, have been found: *FCER2* rs28364072 and *NCOA3* rs2230782. Validation and clinical association studies are needed in order to confirm their pharmacogenomics potential.

Variant *FCER2* rs28364072 is located in the splice-site region and the mutations in that intronic region could influence protein function. Its MAF is around 30% in European populations, but as high as 60% in the population of Africa (**Figure 1**). Therefore, this variant is a candidate pharmacogenomics marker in the African population and further validation and clinical studies are recommended in that population.

The effect of the variant *NCOA3* rs2230782 is probably damaging, according to PolyPhen-2 prediction tool. Its MAF in European population is 10–14% and it is a candidate pharmacogenomics marker in this population. However, MAF for this

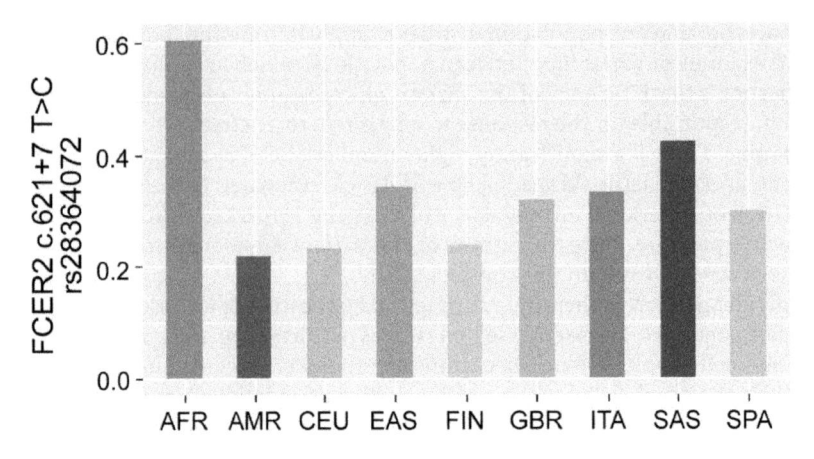

Figure 1.
Distribution of FCER2 rs28364072 MAF in world populations.

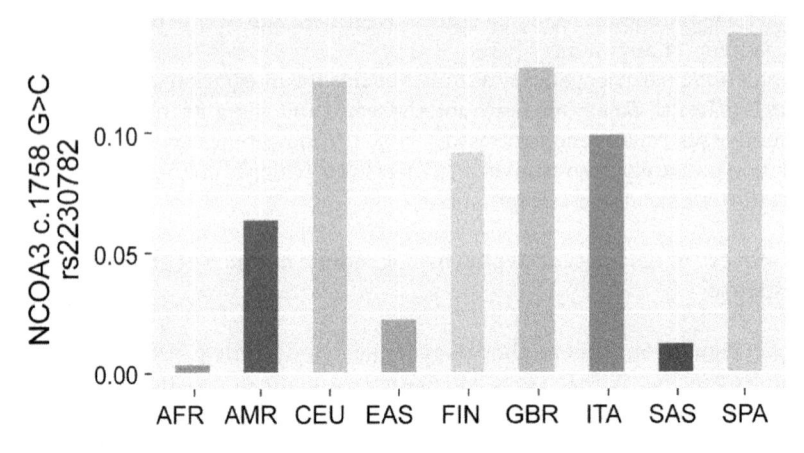

Figure 2.
Distribution of NCOA3 rs2230782 MAF in world populations.

variant is very low in other populations (**Figure 2**). Validation and clinical association studies regarding *NCOA3* rs2230782 pharmacogenomics are recommended only for European populations.

3. Conclusion

Big data in pharmacogenomics and pharmacotranscriptomics was produced so far, but their implementation in clinical practice is poor. Particularly, no pharmacogenomics marker related to GC therapy is reliable enough to be recommended for pre-emptive genetic testing.

A population specific pharmacogenomics landscape relevant for GC therapy could contribute to better understanding of the inconsistency in therapy response and could be helpful in predicting a higher risk of developing adverse reactions in patients that need to be treated with GCs.

Research efforts in the field of pharmacogenomics and pharmacotranscriptomics ought to be directed to data analysis and design of prediction models using machine learning algorithms. Bioinformatics tools and implementation of artificial intelligence are expected to open the door wide for personalized treatment of children with ALL.

Acknowledgements

This work was supported by Ministry of Education, Science and Technological Development Republic of Serbia, EB: 451-03-9/2021-14/200042.

Conflict of interest

The authors declare no conflict of interest.

Abbreviations

ABCB1	ATP binding cassette subfamily B member 1
ALL	Acute lymphoblastic leukemia
BclI	*Bacillus caldolyticus* I restriction enzyme
BFM	Berlin-Frankfurt-Munster
CBG	Corticosteroid binding globulin
CNTNAP2	Contactin-associated protein-like-2
CRHR1	Corticotropin-releasing hormone receptor 1
CRP	C-reactive protein
FDA	Food and Drug Administration
FCER2	Fc Fragment Of IgE Receptor II
G6PD	Glucose-6-phosphate-dehydrogenase
GAS5	Growth arrest-specific 5
GC	Glucocorticoid
GR	Glucocorticoid receptor
GRE	Glucocorticoid response element
GRIK1	Glutamate Ionotropic Receptor Kainate Type Subunit 1
GRIN3A	Glutamate Ionotropic Receptor NMDA Type Subunit 3A
GST	Glutathione S-transferase
GWAS	Genome wide association study
LEPR	Leptin receptor
lncRNA	Long non-coding RNA
MAF	Minor allele frequency
miRNA/miR	Micro RNA
NCBI	National Center for Biotechnology
NCOA3	Nuclear Receptor Coactivator 3
ncRNA	Non-coding RNA
NGS	Next generation sequencing
NR3C1	Nuclear Receptor Subfamily 3 Group C Member 1
PGP	P-glycoprotein
PharmGKB	Pharmacogenomics Knowledge Base
SNP	Single nucleotide polymorphism
VA	Variant annotation

Author details

Vladimir Gasic, Djordje Pavlovic, Biljana Stankovic, Nikola Kotur, Branka Zukic and Sonja Pavlovic*
Institute of Molecular Genetics and Genetic Engineering, University of Belgrade, Belgrade, Serbia

*Address all correspondence to: sonya@imgge.bg.ac.rs

IntechOpen

© 2021 The Author(s). Licensee IntechOpen. This chapter is distributed under the terms of the Creative Commons Attribution License (http://creativecommons.org/licenses/by/3.0), which permits unrestricted use, distribution, and reproduction in any medium, provided the original work is properly cited.

References

[1] Georgitsi M, Zukic B, Pavlovic S, Patrinos GP. Transcriptional regulation and pharmacogenomics. Pharmacogenomics. 2011 May;12(5):655-73.

[2] Stojiljkovic M, P Patrinos G, Pavlovic S. Clinical applicability of sequence variations in genes related to drug metabolism. Current drug metabolism. 2011 Jun 1;12(5):445-54.

[3] FDA. Table of Pharmacogenetic Associations. 2021. Avalialbe from: https://www.fda.gov/medical-devices/precision-medicine/table-pharmacogenetic-associations 05/24/2021

[4] Pui CH, Robison LL, Look AT. Acute lymphoblastic leukaemia. The Lancet. 2008 Mar 22;371(9617):1030-43.

[5] Möricke A, Zimmermann M, Valsecchi MG, Stanulla M, Biondi A, Mann G, Locatelli F, Cazzaniga G, Niggli F, Arico M, Bartram CR. Dexamethasone vs prednisone in induction treatment of pediatric ALL: results of the randomized trial AIEOP-BFM ALL 2000. Blood. 2016 Apr 28;127(17):2101-12.

[6] Gervasini G, Vagace JM. Impact of genetic polymorphisms on chemotherapy toxicity in childhood acute lymphoblastic leukemia. Frontiers in genetics. 2012 Nov 22;3:249.

[7] Hunger SP, Mullighan CG. Acute lymphoblastic leukemia in children. New England Journal of Medicine. 2015 Oct 15;373(16):1541-52.

[8] Pui CH, Pei D, Sandlund JT, Ribeiro RC, Rubnitz JE, Raimondi SC, Onciu M, Campana D, Kun LE, Jeha S, Cheng C. Long-term results of St Jude Total Therapy Studies 11, 12, 13A, 13B, and 14 for childhood acute lymphoblastic leukemia. Leukemia. 2010 Feb;24(2):371-82.

[9] Schrappe M, Reiter A, Ludwig WD, Harbott J, Zimmermann M, Hiddemann W, Niemeyer C, Henze G, Feldges A, Zintl F, Kornhuber B. Improved outcome in childhood acute lymphoblastic leukemia despite reduced use of anthracyclines and cranial radiotherapy: results of trial ALL-BFM 90. Blood, The Journal of the American Society of Hematology. 2000 Jun 1; 95(11):3310-22.

[10] IC-BFM AL. A Randomized Trial of the I-BFM-SG FOR the Management of Childhood non-B acute Lymphoblastic Leukemia. Final Version of Therapy Protocol from August-14-2009. 2009 Aug.

[11] Yang L, Panetta JC, Cai X, Yang W, Pei D, Cheng C, Kornegay N, Pui CH, Relling MV. Asparaginase may influence dexamethasone pharmacokinetics in acute lymphoblastic leukemia. Journal of Clinical Oncology. 2008 Apr 20; 26(12):1932-9.

[12] Pavlovic S, Kotur N, Stankovic B, Zukic B, Gasic V, Dokmanovic L. Pharmacogenomic and pharmacotranscriptomic profiling of childhood acute lymphoblastic leukemia: paving the way to personalized treatment. Genes. 2019 Mar;10(3):191.

[13] Gross KL, Lu NZ, Cidlowski JA. Molecular mechanisms regulating glucocorticoid sensitivity and resistance. Molecular and cellular endocrinology. 2009 Mar 5;300(1-2):7-16.

[14] Tissing WJ, Meijerink JP, den Boer ML, Brinkhof B, van Rossum EF, van Wering ER, Koper JW, Sonneveld P, Pieters R. Genetic variations in the glucocorticoid receptor gene are not related to glucocorticoid resistance in childhood acute lymphoblastic leukemia. Clinical cancer research. 2005 Aug 15;11(16):6050-6.

[15] Huizenga NA, Koper JW, de Lange P, Pols HA, Stolk RP, Burger H,

Grobbee DE, Brinkmann AO, de Jong FH, Lamberts SW. A polymorphism in the glucocorticoid receptor gene may be associated with an increased sensitivity to glucocorticoids in vivo. The Journal of Clinical Endocrinology & Metabolism. 1998 Jan 1;83(1):144-51.

[16] Feng J, Zheng J, Bennett WP, Heston LL, Jones IR, Craddock N, Sommer SS. Five missense variants in the amino-terminal domain of the glucocorticoid receptor: No association with puerperal psychosis or schizophrenia. American journal of medical genetics. 2000 Jun 12;96(3):412-7.

[17] Jewell CM, Cidlowski JA. Molecular evidence for a link between the N363S glucocorticoid receptor polymorphism and altered gene expression. The Journal of Clinical Endocrinology & Metabolism. 2007 Aug 1;92(8):3268-77.

[18] Eipel OT, Németh K, Török D, Csordas K, Hegyi M, Ponyi A, Ferenczy A, Erdélyi DJ, Csóka M, Kovács GT. The glucocorticoid receptor gene polymorphism N363S predisposes to more severe toxic side effects during pediatric acute lymphoblastic leukemia (ALL) therapy. International journal of hematology. 2013 Feb;97(2):216-22.

[19] Van Rossum EF, Koper JW, Van Den Beld AW, Uitterlinden AG, Arp P, Ester W, Janssen JA, Brinkmann AO, De Jong FH, Grobbee DE, Pols HA. Identification of the BclI polymorphism in the glucocorticoid receptor gene: association with sensitivity to glucocorticoids in vivo and body mass index. Clinical endocrinology. 2003 Nov;59(5):585-92.

[20] Xue LU, Li C, Wang Y, Sun W, Ma C, He Y, Yu Y, Cai L, Wang L. Single nucleotide polymorphisms in noncoding region of the glucocorticoid receptor gene and prednisone response in childhood acute lymphoblastic leukemia. Leukemia & lymphoma. 2015 Jun 3;56(6):1704-9.

[21] Stevens A, Ray DW, Zeggini E, John S, Richards HL, Griffiths CE, Donn R. Glucocorticoid sensitivity is determined by a specific glucocorticoid receptor haplotype. The Journal of Clinical Endocrinology & Metabolism. 2004 Feb 1;89(2):892-7.

[22] Van Rossum EF, Roks PH, De Jong FH, Brinkmann AO, Pols HA, Koper JW, Lamberts SW. Characterization of a promoter polymorphism in the glucocorticoid receptor gene and its relationship to three other polymorphisms. Clinical endocrinology. 2004 Nov;61(5):573-81.

[23] Russcher H, van Rossum EF, de Jong FH, Brinkmann AO, Lamberts SW, Koper JW. Increased expression of the glucocorticoid receptor-A translational isoform as a result of the ER22/23EK polymorphism. Molecular Endocrinology. 2005 Jul 1;19(7):1687-96.

[24] Derijk RH, Schaaf MJ, Turner GO, Datson NA, Vreugdenhil ER, Cidlowski JO, de Kloet ER, Emery PA, Sternberg EM, Detera-Wadleigh SD. A human glucocorticoid receptor gene variant that increases the stability of the glucocorticoid receptor beta-isoform mRNA is associated with rheumatoid arthritis. The Journal of rheumatology. 2001 Nov 1;28(11):2383-8.

[25] Gasic V, Zukic B, Stankovic B, Janic D, Dokmanovic L, Lazic J, Krstovski N, Dolzan V, Jazbec J, Pavlovic S, Kotur N. Pharmacogenomic markers of glucocorticoid response in the initial phase of remission induction therapy in childhood acute lymphoblastic leukemia. Radiology and oncology. 2018 Sep;52(3):296.

[26] Farrell RJ, Menconi MJ, Keates AC, Kelly CP. P-glycoprotein-170 inhibition significantly reduces cortisol and ciclosporin efflux from human intestinal

epithelial cells and T lymphocytes. Alimentary pharmacology & therapeutics. 2002 May;16(5):1021-31.

[27] Hoffmeyer SO, Burk O, Von Richter O, Arnold HP, Brockmöller J, Johne A, Cascorbi I, Gerloff T, Roots I, Eichelbaum M, Brinkmann U. Functional polymorphisms of the human multidrug-resistance gene: multiple sequence variations and correlation of one allele with P-glycoprotein expression and activity in vivo. Proceedings of the National Academy of Sciences. 2000 Mar 28;97(7):3473-8.

[28] Wang D, Johnson AD, Papp AC, Kroetz DL, Sadee W. Multidrug resistance polypeptide 1 (MDR1, ABCB1) variant 3435C> T affects mRNA stability. Pharmacogenetics and genomics. 2005 Oct 1;15(10):693-704.

[29] Kimchi-Sarfaty C, Oh JM, Kim IW, Sauna ZE, Calcagno AM, Ambudkar SV, Gottesman MM. A" silent" polymorphism in the MDR1 gene changes substrate specificity. Science. 2007 Jan 26;315(5811):525-8.

[30] Jamroziak K, Młynarski W, Balcerczak E, Mistygacz M, Treliṅska J, Mirowski M, Bodalski J, Robak T. Functional C3435T polymorphism of MDR1 gene: an impact on genetic susceptibility and clinical outcome of childhood acute lymphoblastic leukemia. European journal of haematology. 2004 May;72(5):314-21.

[31] Gregers J, Green H, Christensen IJ, Dalhoff K, Schroeder H, Carlsen N, Rosthoej S, Lausen B, Schmiegelow K, Peterson C. Polymorphisms in the ABCB1 gene and effect on outcome and toxicity in childhood acute lymphoblastic leukemia. The pharmacogenomics journal. 2015 Aug;15(4):372-9.

[32] Crouthamel MH, Wu D, Yang Z, Ho RJ. A novel MDR1 G1199T variant alters drug resistance and efflux transport activity of P-glycoprotein in recombinant Hek cells. Journal of pharmaceutical sciences. 2006 Dec 1;95(12):2767-77.

[33] Homma H, Listowsky I. Identification of Yb-glutathione-S-transferase as a major rat liver protein labeled with dexamethasone 21-methanesulfonate. Proceedings of the National Academy of Sciences. 1985 Nov 1;82(21):7165-9.

[34] Anderer G, Schrappe M, Brechlin AM, Lauten M, Muti P, Welte K, Stanulla M. Polymorphisms within glutathione S-transferase genes and initial response to glucocorticoids in childhood acute lymphoblastic leukaemia. Pharmacogenetics and Genomics. 2000 Nov 1;10(8):715-26.

[35] Takanashi M, Morimoto A, Yagi T, Kuriyama K, Kano G, Imamura T, Hibi S, Todo S, Imashuku S. Impact of glutathione S-transferase gene deletion on early relapse in childhood B-precursor acute lymphoblastic leukemia. Haematologica. 2003 Jan 1;88(11):1238-44.

[36] Franca R, Rebora P, Basso G, Biondi A, Cazzaniga G, Crovella S, Decorti G, Fagioli F, Giarin E, Locatelli F, Poggi V. Glutathione S-transferase homozygous deletions and relapse in childhood acute lymphoblastic leukemia: a novel study design in a large Italian AIEOP cohort. Pharmacogenomics. 2012 Dec;13(16):1905-16.

[37] Davies SM, Bhatia S, Ross JA, Kiffmeyer WR, Gaynon PS, Radloff GA, Robison LL, Perentesis JP. Glutathione S-transferase genotypes, genetic susceptibility, and outcome of therapy in childhood acute lymphoblastic leukemia. Blood, The Journal of the American Society of Hematology. 2002 Jul 1;100(1):67-71.

[38] Johansson AS, Stenberg G, Widersten M, Mannervik B. Structure-activity relationships and thermal stability of human glutathione

transferase P1-1 governed by the H-site residue 105. Journal of molecular biology. 1998 May 8;278(3):687-98.

[39] Jackson RK, Irving JA, Veal GJ. Personalization of dexamethasone therapy in childhood acute lymphoblastic leukaemia. British journal of haematology. 2016 Apr;173(1):13-24.

[40] Kamdem LK, Hamilton L, Cheng C, Liu W, Yang W, Johnson JA, Pui CH, Relling MV. Genetic predictors of glucocorticoid-induced hypertension in children with acute lymphoblastic leukemia. Pharmacogenetics and genomics. 2008 Jun 1;18(6):507-14.

[41] Karol SE, Yang W, Van Driest SL, Chang TY, Kaste S, Bowton E, Basford M, Bastarache L, Roden DM, Denny JC, Larsen E. Genetics of glucocorticoid-associated osteonecrosis in children with acute lymphoblastic leukemia. Blood, The Journal of the American Society of Hematology. 2015 Oct 8;126(15):1770-6.

[42] Bolton JL, Hayward C, Direk N, Lewis JG, Hammond GL, Hill LA, Anderson A, Huffman J, Wilson JF, Campbell H, Rudan I. Genome wide association identifies common variants at the SERPINA6/SERPINA1 locus influencing plasma cortisol and corticosteroid binding globulin. PLoS Genet. 2014 Jul 10;10(7):e1004474.

[43] Yang JJ, Cheng C, Devidas M, Cao X, Campana D, Yang W, Fan Y, Neale G, Cox N, Scheet P, Borowitz MJ. Genome-wide association study identifies germline polymorphisms associated with relapse of childhood acute lymphoblastic leukemia. Blood, The Journal of the American Society of Hematology. 2012 Nov 15;120(20):4197-204.

[44] Gasic V, Stankovic B, Zukic B, Janic D, Dokmanovic L, Krstovski N, Lazic J, Milosevic G, Lucafò M, Stocco G, Decorti G. Expression pattern of long non-coding RNA growth arrest-specific 5 in the remission induction therapy in childhood acute lymphoblastic leukemia. Journal of medical biochemistry. 2019 Jul;38(3):292.

[45] Kino T, Hurt DE, Ichijo T, Nader N, Chrousos GP. Noncoding RNA gas5 is a growth arrest–and starvation-associated repressor of the glucocorticoid receptor. Science signaling. 2010 Feb 2;3(107):ra8-.

[46] Chen H, Zhang D, Zhang G, Li X, Liang Y, Kasukurthi MV, Li S, Borchert GM, Huang J. A semantics-oriented computational approach to investigate microRNA regulation on glucocorticoid resistance in pediatric acute lymphoblastic leukemia. BMC medical informatics and decision making. 2018 Jul;18(2):149-57.

[47] Lv M, Zhang X, Jia H, Li D, Zhang B, Zhang H, Hong M, Jiang T, Jiang Q, Lu J, Huang X. An oncogenic role of miR-142-3p in human T-cell acute lymphoblastic leukemia (T-ALL) by targeting glucocorticoid receptor-α and cAMP/PKA pathways. Leukemia. 2012 Apr;26(4):769-77.

[48] Harada M, Pokrovskaja-Tamm K, Söderhäll S, Heyman M, Grander D, Corcoran M. Involvement of miR17 pathway in glucocorticoid-induced cell death in pediatric acute lymphoblastic leukemia. Leukemia & lymphoma. 2012 Oct 1;53(10):2041-50.

[49] Stanković B, Kotur N, Gašić V, Klaassen K, Ristivojević B, Stojiljković M, Pavlović S, Zukić B. Pharmacogenomics landscape of COVID-19 therapy response in Serbian population and comparison with worldwide populations. Journal of medical biochemistry. 2020 Oct 2;39(4):488.

[50] Whirl-Carrillo M, McDonagh EM, Hebert JM, Gong L, Sangkuhl K, Thorn CF, Altman RB, Klein TE.

Pharmacogenomics knowledge for personalized medicine. Clinical Pharmacology & Therapeutics. 2012 Oct;92(4):414-7.

[51] Engen RM, Marsh S, Van Booven DJ, McLeod HL. Ethnic differences in pharmacogenetically relevant genes. Current drug targets. 2006 Dec 1;7(12):1641-8.

[52] Carson PE, Flanagan CL, Ickes CE, Alving AS. Enzymatic deficiency in primaquine-sensitive erythrocytes. Science. 1956 Sep 14;124(3220):484-5.

[53] Mette L, Mitropoulos K, Vozikis A, Patrinos GP. Pharmacogenomics and public health: implementing 'populationalized'medicine. Pharmacogenomics. 2012 May;13(7):803-13.

[54] Viennas E, Komianou A, Mizzi C, Stojiljkovic M, Mitropoulou C, Muilu J, Vihinen M, Grypioti P, Papadaki S, Pavlidis C, Zukic B. Expanded national database collection and data coverage in the FINDbase worldwide database for clinically relevant genomic variation allele frequencies. Nucleic acids research. 2016 Oct 17:gkw949.

Chapter 5

Corticosteroids in Neuro-Oncology: Management of Intracranial Tumors and Peritumoral Edema

Sunbul S. Ahmed

Abstract

Corticosteroids have been in use for decades and are one of the most prescribed drugs in all specialties of medicine. Jerome Posner, in his classic textbook "Neurological Complications of Cancer," refers to corticosteroids as widely used drugs in neuro-oncology leading to a remarkable decline in perioperative mortality and morbidity rates. Being the most powerful class of tumor-induced-edema reducing agents, they are adjuvant to chemotherapy and are also known to reduce the risk of encephalopathy and other associated neurological deficits in patients undergoing radiation therapy. They have been widely used in higher-than-normal doses in the management of pathologic, immunological, and inflammatory conditions and various other diseases. Novel insights into the mechanisms of action of corticosteroids and their effects on cancer patients are extensively being studied. While substantial clinical improvements can be seen in cancer patients, corticosteroids are also associated with adverse and well-characterized side effects leading to immediate as well as long-term complications in patients. This chapter reviews the clinical aspects of corticosteroid therapy used in neuro-oncological conditions and its effects on peritumoral edema. Although there is currently insufficient information on appropriate use, in most cases, corticosteroids are used in a supraphysiological and pharmacological manner to minimize the symptoms of cerebral edema. Due to limited clinical studies and evident side effects presenting synonymously with corticosteroid therapy, the emerging role of steroid-sparing drugs such as corticotrophin-releasing factors, tyrosine kinase inhibitors, and VEGF inhibitors will also be discussed.

Keywords: Neuro-oncology, brain tumor, cerebral edema, corticosteroid therapy, dexamethasone, bevacizumab

1. Introduction

Corticosteroids are synthetic analogs of a class of naturally synthesized hormone molecules in the adrenal cortex that act as biological mediators. These hormones play a vital role in regulating essential bodily processes such as metabolism, inflammation, response to stress, and electrolyte balance.

Corticosteroids have been classified based on major effects exhibited by them into glucocorticoids and mineralocorticoids. Glucocorticoids provide anti-inflammatory responses by suppressing inflammation and immunity, exert vasoconstrictive, and are responsible for the breakdown of fats, proteins, and carbohydrates. Cortisol is a physiological mediator well-characterized to exhibit glucocorticoid effects in humans. Mineralocorticoids exhibit salt-retaining and electrolyte-balancing properties. A prominent hormone, aldosterone, projects the strongest mineralocorticoid activity. The pioneering of corticosteroids (such as dexamethasone, prednisolone, prednisone) has revolutionized the treatment approaches in the field of clinical oncology [1]. They mimic the action of naturally occurring hormones, are currently one of the most prescribed drugs worldwide, and can be used to treat several conditions such as infections, inflammatory disorders, allergic and autoimmune diseases, shock, lowering of excessive blood calcium levels, hypoglycemia, suppression of excess secretion from the adrenal cortex, prevention of graft rejection, neurological disorders, hematologic disorders, skin disorders, and corticosteroid replacement therapy [2, 3].

Steroids administered to brain tumor patients do not directly treat the tumor but are targeted to reduce edema surrounding the tumor (induced by the tumor itself or its treatment) thereby the mass effect and lymphoma in the central nervous system, prevent or alleviate the symptoms of nausea, vomiting and headache post-chemotherapy and temporarily improve other associated neurological symptoms [1]. They can cross the blood–brain barrier and act as analgesic agents by inhibiting the synthesis of prostaglandins thereby reducing inflammation and tissue edema is resolved by decreasing vascular permeability. Sustained use in high doses requires close monitoring to prevent and manage its side effects and intervene if other complications arise.

2. Traditional approaches to steroid therapy in brain tumor patients

The introduction of steroids, 50 years ago, revolutionized therapeutic approaches in Clinical oncology. The first use of cortisone to treat cerebral edema developed in patients post neurosurgery was accomplished by Ingraham in 1952 [4]. About five years later, Kofman pioneered the use of prednisone for peritumoral edema induced in patients with intracranial malignancies [5]. Dexamethasone, synthesized in 1958, is based on Galcich's experimental demonstration of brain tumor inhibition upon administering large doses of dexamethasone [6]. Its pioneering fundamentally changed the course of corticosteroid therapy in cancer patients and to date has been the most commendable drug due to its conducive effects in alleviating symptoms of tumor-induced cerebral edema and offers benefits of low sodium and water retention index thereby reducing the risk of electrolyte imbalance, low mineralocorticoid effect, and high glucocorticoid potency [1, 7, 8].

With further advancements, exhibited antineoplastic effects of dexamethasone, prednisone, prednisolone, and methylprednisolone against hematologic malignancies, their antiedema, and anti-lymphoma properties were known [9]. The administration of steroids has proved beneficial in rapidly relieving symptoms, minimizing tumor-associated pain, nausea, and vomiting, and ameliorate appetite in tumor patients [10]. Its advantageous characteristics have found immense clinical applications such as in treating patients with carcinomatous meningitis and lymphoma in the central nervous system [11].

3. Molecular mechanisms

Corticosteroids are the mainstay of treatment for neuro-oncological conditions, and they undergo various molecular mechanisms at the cellular level to give desired clinical results. These mechanisms are complex and distinct and with currently limited evidence, are divided into genomic and non-genomic. The consensus is that the genetic level, effects such as an increased rate of transcription known as transactivation, a transrepression-a process in which one protein represses the activity of the second protein, and post-translational regulation i.e., controlling the levels of active protein, can be seen, constituting the genomic mechanism, and producing anti-inflammatory effects. Activating a cascade of signaling pathways constitutes the non-genomic effects. These mechanisms mediate several side-effects, such as diabetes and glaucoma due to transactivation while suppression of hypothalamic–adrenal–pituitary axis due to transactivation. Both transactivation and transrepression seem to be involved in osteoporosis. Glucocorticoids bind to complementary cytoplasmic receptors upon diffusion through the plasma membrane. The binding of this free glucocorticoid receptor leads to the release of a heat-shock protein 90 kDa which in turn exposes two nuclear localization signals responsible for facilitating the movement of the glucocorticoid–receptor complex into the nucleus [12]. Specific DNA (deoxyribonucleic acid) elements called glucocorticoid response elements (GRE) regulate the transcription of nuclear DNA. Synthesis of several cytokines and chemokines involved in regulating inflammatory reactions such as *eotaxin* and *lipocortin 1* is suppressed by glucocorticoids at the level of transcription [13]. The interaction of glucocorticoids with other transcription factors such as p53 indirectly influences their activity on their target genes [14]. The production of proinflammatory cytokines and chemokines is controlled by transcription factors such as NF-КB, CRE-binding proteins, among others, and leads to activation of inflammatory pathways. Therefore, inhibiting these transcription factors induces anti-inflammatory responses [12, 15]. To summarize the mechanism: corticosteroids bind to intracellular cytoplasmic receptors upon crossing the plasma membrane and form the steroid–receptor complex. Consequently, the movement of the steroid-receptor complex into the nucleus directly influences the transcription of genes and upon interaction with other transcription factors, a non-transcriptional regulation of other signaling cascades is mediated.

4. Vasogenic edema and Antiedema property of corticosteroids

The use of corticosteroids for the management of malignant brain tumors and symptomatic peritumoral edema was recognized several decades ago [3]. They are frequently prescribed to reduce the increased intracranial pressure caused due to peritumoral fluid accumulation. Although edema occurs in patients with malignant lesions but is also evident in cases of benign tumors such as meningiomas [16, 17]. A disruption in the blood–brain barrier leads to the flow of fluid into extracellular spaces of brain parenchyma resulting in vasogenic edema. This disruption results in increased permeability of the BBB primarily due to the opening of the inter-endothelial tight junctions and increased endothelial pinocytosis and endothelial fenestrations [18, 19]. An insufficient number of normal astrocytes, responsible for producing factors that are required for the formation of normal BBB, results in defects in endothelial tight junctions, production of cytokines such as vascular endothelial growth factor (VEGF) [20], and hepatocyte growth factor [21] by both benign and malignant brain tumors and increase tumor vessel permeability [22]. The suggested mechanism of corticosteroids is a reduction in permeability of tumor vessels by upregulation of genes and molecules such as occludin, a tight junction component in endothelial cells [23], and by dephosphorylating occludin and another TJ component, zona occludens (ZO1) [24]. Another mechanism of influencing the endothelial permeability is by non-transcriptional regulation of capillaries that involves rearranging and attachment of vascular endothelial (VE)-cadherin to the cytoskeleton [25]. The permeability of the blood–brain barrier is decreased upon steroid administration and this limits the extravasation of fluids [26, 27].

5. Treatment of Lymphomatous neoplasms

Steroids are frequently prescribed in patients with primary lymphoma in the central nervous system or in cases of secondary lymphomatous neoplasms where they rapidly respond by promoting cell cycle arrest and cell death by the mechanism of apoptosis in a p38 mitogen-activated protein kinase (MAPK) dependent manner in B and T cells [27–29]. Steroids are administered during the initial stages along with chemotherapy and the clinical and radiographic response can be rapid in cases of lymphoma and inflammatory conditions. Some preclinical studies suggest that proliferation of some glioma cells may reduce upon dexamethasone exposure [30]. On the other hand, certain reports suggest that steroids have no effect or stimulate the growth of glioma cells [31, 32]. Effects of steroids can be transient and require chemotherapy or irradiation to prevent the recurrence of the tumor [33]. Furthermore, there is no significant clinical evidence so far that proves the role of steroids in the growth inhibition of gliomas or metastasis in humans.

6. Anti-emetic properties

Steroids are administered either singly or in combination with 5HT-3 receptor antagonists, neurokinin-1 receptor antagonists, and aprepitant for the prophylaxis and the treatment of chemotherapy-induced nausea and vomiting and to manage subsequent symptoms of dehydration and electrolyte imbalance [34]. Steroid administration leads to a reduced release of serotonin from hematocytes and this directly affects the cellular expression of its receptors, thereby preventing nausea and vomiting [35, 36]. The most favorable corticosteroids are methylprednisolone and dexamethasone in patients with moderate to high emetogenic chemotherapy.

7. Dosing and tapering

Steroid administration is adjuvant to chemotherapy and all cancer patients will receive steroid therapy at some point in their cancer treatment and may continue to receive them through surgery, chemotherapy, radiation, and prolonged use may be needed because of its benefits of symptomatic relief. Despite its extensive use, there is a lack of significant clinical evidence about the choice of drug, dose, duration, and tapering schemes.

Various clinical trials have been conducted that aim to assess the effects of doses of 8 mg versus 16 mg dexamethasone and 4 mg versus 16 mg in patients with peritumoral edema. Significant clinical improvement among all groups administered with dexamethasone can be seen on the Karnofsky performance scale. Low doses of dexamethasone (4-8 mg/day) are recommended to avoid developing serious complications but they may require reinstitution after cessation of steroid therapy [37]. Whereas higher doses of dexamethasone (16 mg/day) along with osmotherapy (mannitol, glycerol) or surgery, may be required in adverse conditions [38]. In some cases, higher than usual doses may be required for headaches. Current evidence has a lack of information about the correlation between dose and body weight or dose and age. Attempts to standardize the steroid therapy regimen have remained unsuccessful and it is suggested that the dosage must be altered according to the specific needs of the patient depending on the size of the lesion, location, mass effect, and presenting symptoms. It is recommended that for successful results and for preventing steroid-associated toxicity, tapering should be considered as soon as clinically acceptable [39]. Interestingly, a longer duration of 23 weeks of steroid therapy is required for patients with a primary brain tumor as opposed to 7 weeks that is required for secondary brain tumors. Steroid therapy can be stopped quickly in patients that have been receiving it for a shorter duration, usually 10–14 days. On the other hand, careful and closely monitored tapering is required for patients with prolonged steroid use to avoid declination of their medical state and/or dependency or withdrawal effects and evident hypercortisolism. Hydrocortisone, which is commonly prescribed in 2 doses per day to mimic the physiological action of cortisol in patients with its deficient levels. 20 mg and 10 mg dose administration in the morning and afternoon, respectively, are suggested for patients with remarkably high cortisol insufficiency [40].

8. Side effects

Depending on the type of drug and prescribed dose, a wide spectrum of systemic and neurological side effects can occur in response to corticosteroid therapy. While manifestations of some side effects can be seen immediately upon administration of corticosteroids, others may develop over time and may persist even after steroid therapy has been terminated, such as cataract formation and osteoporosis [1]. Most side effects are easily manageable, but some can be fatal. Patients considered at substantial risk have impaired immune systems either due to organ transplantation or upon undergoing chemotherapy or radiotherapy.

8.1 Systemic

Systemic side effects include a cushingoid appearance, truncal obesity, hirsutism, acne, impaired wound healing, striae, nausea, anorexia, easy bruising and capillary fragility, immunosuppression, hypertension, increased risk of infections, respiratory muscle weakness, glucose intolerance, electrolyte disturbance, fluid retention, peripheral edema, increased appetite, gastrointestinal bleeding, growth retardation, cataracts, glaucoma, and visual blurring [41].

Arterial hypertension, considered as the most common side effect, occurs in 20% of the patients. It is usually reversible and blood pressure values attain a normal value upon cessation of steroid intake. For patients whose steroid therapy cannot be discontinued, hypertension requires symptomatic treatment. Since the main cause of hypertension is an abnormal increase in the volume of blood plasma by steroids, the preferred line of treatment is the use of diuretics [42].

8.2 Gastrointestinal

Although, no significant correlation between steroid usage and gastrointestinal bleeding has been found in clinical studies, yet histamine H2 antagonists and proton pump inhibitors are commonly prescribed to minimize the risk of gastric ulcers, hemorrhage, and other rare gastrointestinal problems such as pancreatitis, colon perforation, and fatty liver disease [43–45].

8.3 Osteoporosis

An increase in cases of developing osteoporosis and avascular necrosis is seen in patients receiving steroid therapy evident from the lumbar spine and hip fractures [46, 47]. Although several factors can contribute to the occurrence of osteoporosis, yet the suggested mechanism is that due to skeletal muscles getting directly affected by the glucocorticoids, calcium absorption is reduced leading to hyperparathyroidism and a decrease in gonadal hormones. Molecular studies suggest a decrease in IGH-1 and prostaglandin E2, which are responsible for stimulating bone growth [48]. Administration of phenytoin and valproic acid also promote osteoporosis [49–51]. To prevent/manage the symptoms of osteoporosis calcium supplements (1500 mg/day), Vitamin D (800 international units/day) [48], and bisphosphonates such as alendronate and zoledronate are commonly prescribed [52]. Kyphoplasty may be required in patients with severe pain from compression fractions.

8.4 Neurological and neuropsychiatric

Common neurological side effects of corticosteroids are myopathy, visual blurring, tremor, behavioral changes, headache, reduced taste and smell, and cerebral atrophy while rare complications include psychosis, hallucinations, neck flexors, dementia, seizures, dependency, epidural lipomatosis, and neuropathy.

Most pervasive yet mild neuropsychiatric effects such as anxiety, insomnia, irritability, euphoria, and mood disturbances may develop in response to corticosteroid therapy. Adverse effects include euphoria, steroid-induced dementia, cortical atrophy, cognitive dysfunction, memory loss, and psychotic episodes that may occur but are more likely in patients with a history of psychiatric disorders. Episodes of seizures may relapse in patients with a history of seizure disorder. Impairment in physiology during the development of the brain such as hippocampal neurogenesis is seen in animal models administered with corticosteroids. Similarly, prednisolone has been shown to negatively affect verbal memory function in humans and long-term cognitive dysfunction is evident in children if taken in combination with dexamethasone. However, it can be challenging to differentiate between the manifestations of radiation therapy, gliomas, and the increase in levels of intracranial pressure with complications occurring due to corticosteroid use. Discontinuation or tapering is recommended for managing steroid-induced neuropsychiatric effects as soon as clinically acceptable. Prednisone dose must be kept lower than 40 mg/day. The use of Neuroleptics, valproic acid, and lithium can be considered but tricyclic antidepressants should be avoided as they can worsen the condition [53–57].

8.5 Myopathy

Although the pathophysiology of steroid myopathy remains unknown, yet it has been shown to negatively affect the quality of life in patients. Clinical studies suggest that steroid myopathy occurs more commonly (almost 10%) in patients with primary brain tumors administered with fluorinated glucocorticoids such as dexamethasone over the ones administered with non-fluorinated glucocorticoids, such as hydrocortisone or prednisone (which may not have proven to be highly effective in controlling cerebral edema) [58–60]. Common symptoms associated with steroid myopathy are a proximal weakness with normal sensation and deep tendon reflexes intact. Detection is made using electromyography. The probable mechanism of steroid myopathy can be protein synthesis inhibition, increased protein catabolism, and induction of the activity of glutamine synthetase [61, 62]. Development of muscle weakness may develop even upon administration of low doses over a shorter duration and may not occur in patients even with high doses and prolonged duration of application. Individuals without symptoms of myopathy may also be considered at minimal risk for developing cushingoid features and fluid retention. In patients with steroid myopathy, the accepted standard of management is the cessation of steroids, but it may still require months for recovery to take place. Steroid-induced muscle wasting is demonstrated to be reduced by muscle activity and hence exercise and muscle therapy are recommended to alleviate the symptoms or reduce the risk of developing steroid myopathy [63].

8.6 Adrenal insufficiency (AI)

About 1% of patients receiving steroid therapy for the treatment of brain tumors develop steroid adrenal insufficiency upon sudden glucocorticoid withdrawal. The presenting symptoms of AI are like those of increased intracranial pressure and side effects of antineoplastic treatment. Management of AI is focused on hydrocortisone treatment and dosage is similar to that recommended for other major surgeries [64].

8.7 Diabetes

Diabetes occurs in up to 50% of steroid-treated patients and is the most common form of drug-induced diabetes mellitus [65]. It is already well known that corticosteroids, such as dexamethasone, prednisone, and hydrocortisone, cause elevations in blood glucose levels in both patients regardless of pre-existing diabetes. Severe hyperglycemia may lead to acute or severe complications, such as dehydration, impaired immune system and wound healing, increased risk of infection, ketoacidosis, and acute hyperglycemic syndrome. According to the Joint British Diabetes Association (JBDA), the predisposing factors for steroid-induced hyperglycemia as pre-existing type 1 or 2 diabetes, obesity, family history of diabetes, among others. Management of steroid-induced diabetes is similar to that of regular type 2 diabetes, and patients consistently showing high blood sugar levels should be treated to prevent long-term complications including cardiovascular and renal damage.

8.8 Steroid withdrawal

Continued corticosteroid therapy can be recommended for patients with advanced or terminal diseases or those in hospice care to prevent withdrawal symptoms including those of steroid-pseudo rheumatism, myalgia, abdominal pain, nausea, arthralgia, and acute adrenal insufficiency (highest risk with more than 6 weeks of administration). The occurrence of these complications with corticosteroid discontinuation would require further medication and treatment, aggravating the symptoms of restlessness, excessive sleepiness and can act as contributing factors in relapsing of masked symptoms. It must be noted that continued corticosteroid administration would still require managing its side effects such as insomnia, hypertension, hyperglycemia, and psychotic episodes.

9. Immunological response to corticosteroids

Immunosuppression is common in response to dexamethasone causing inhibition of immune and inflammatory responses and therefore, posing a challenge for the development of immunotherapeutic approaches in late-stage cancer treatment. Risk of life-threatening fungal infections such as *Pneumocystis jirovecii* is elevated with administration of moderate to high doses [66].

While the exact mechanism is unknown, dexamethasone has been shown to promote apoptosis in T-lymphocytes [67], suggesting directive nature of T-cell positive and negative selection in the thymus by glucocorticoids, limiting the activation-induced cell death during the contraction phase of an adaptive immune response and induction of generalized thymocyte apoptosis after polyclonal T-cell activation [68]. A shift in immune response towards a Th2 humoral response from a Th1 cellular response is induced by influencing the levels of cytokines produced by the lymphocytes [69]. Moreover, dexamethasone causes a reduction in the number of splenic and lymph node B-cells and attenuation of early B-cell progenitor proliferation. Glucocorticoids also enhance the activity of macrophages and promote tolerance in dendritic cells thereby, exerting a potent anti-inflammatory effect [70]. The risk for infection may increase by steroid-induced lymphopenia but it also limits the number of treatment strategies applied for activating the immune system and boosting anti-tumor responses.

10. Immunotherapy

Novel immunotherapeutic agents such as ipilimumab are proving their potential efficacy in the treatment of malignant gliomas. A studied mechanism is that it targets cytotoxic T lymphocyte-associated antigen 4 and interferes with the inhibition of T-cell function, which subsequently translates into enhanced antitumor activity.

Current clinical developments are focusing on programmed cell death of immune cell receptor. Hence, clinical trials are being conducted on ipilimumab, that contains anti-programmed cell death-1 antibody, nivolumab for the treatment of glioblastoma [71, 72]. Steroids may interfere with boosting immune response and therefore can be counterproductive for patients delivered with vaccines. Accordingly, several vaccination trials restrict the use of steroids at the time of enrollment to select only patients with a suitable immunological profile.

11. Dexamethasone and phenytoin interactions

Phenytoin is prescribed prophylactically before surgery and in combination with dexamethasone during the initial stages of primary and secondary metastatic brain tumors. Phenytoin may exert protective effects in reducing the risk of steroid-induced myopathy, but the mechanism remains unclear. It is suggested that an increase in the rate of metabolic clearance of cortisol and dexamethasone by phenytoin and decrease in half-life of dexamethasone by 50% and its metabolic conversion to hydroxyl metabolite by the action of CYP3A4, a liver enzyme could be the probable mechanism [73–76]. Levels of phenytoin are contrastingly altered upon co-administration with dexamethasone [77–79]. Hence it is difficult to measure levels of phenytoin in patients taking dexamethasone. Therefore, it also becomes extremely important to carefully monitor levels of phenytoin and tapering should be done as soon as the edema is successfully controlled [80].

12. Dexamethasone and chemotherapy

Administration of glucocorticoids may significantly contribute to altering the pharmacokinetics and may restrict the action of chemotherapeutic drugs from exerting the blood–brain barrier, therefore, limiting the desired effects. It was hypothesized by Duan et al., that hyperglycemia (occurring in response to corticosteroid therapy) inhibits apoptosis and therefore promotes malignant growth, causing proliferation of cells, speeding up the process of metastasis, and aiding resistance to chemotherapy. Dexamethasone exerts protective effects against apoptotic action of temozolomide in glioma cells in vitro [81]. Ongoing experiments aim to determine the antagonizing or synergizing action of dexamethasone with chemotherapeutic drugs such as rapamycin and apoptotic drugs like staurosporine. Pretreatment and subsequent cotreatment strategies for experiments have indicated an additive effect of dexamethasone in combination with growth factor signaling inhibitors.

13. Alternatives to corticosteroids

Steroids have been shown to have limited effects of clinical significance and there are several side effects associated with it. Therefore, a need for novel anti-angiogenic alternatives such as Bevacizumab with strong steroid-sparing, more effective, and less toxic characteristics, arises. It is a neutralizing antibody that targets a specific protein called VEGF, responsible for promoting the growth and spread of tumor blood vessels, therefore reducing peritumoral edema. A major challenge in the action of anti-VEGF is the inhibition of the action of other drugs administered to target the tumor since drugs similar to bevacizumab also affect normal blood vessels. An approval for bevacizumab is still lacking and the cost is a barrier. Other similar drugs are VEGF -receptor inhibitors such as cediranib, sorafenib, sunitinib. In the same way, tyrosine kinase inhibitors (TKIs) such as cediranib and cabozantinib, target vascular endothelial growth factor receptor 2 (VEGFR-2). Similarly, drugs such as corticorelin acetate, a synthetic analog of corticotropin-releasing factor have been proved to reduce edema by directly acting on CR1 and CR2 receptors in animal models and allows higher maximal reduction of the dexamethasone dose compared with control-treated brain tumor patients in a randomized trial [82–84]. Also, patients receiving corticorelin acetate are less likely to be affected by myopathy or cushingoid appearance. There are still undergoing trials to determine its efficacy in acute and chronic peritumoral edema. The effects of other drugs such as boswellic acids, cyclooxygenase (COX)-2 inhibitors, and angiotensin-II inhibitors on brain tumors is still uncertain [85–87].

14. Glucose levels in patients administered with corticosteroids

Corticosteroid use may cause hyperglycemia in almost 20–50% of patients, therefore negatively affecting patient outcomes. A study conducted in Sunnybrook Odette Cancer Centre in Toronto and published in Annals of Palliative Medicine, upon categorizing patients with and without pre-existing diabetes according to the Canadian Diabetes Association (CDA) criterion for diagnosis of diabetes, concluded that the effects of corticosteroids are dose-dependent and tend to impact random plasma glucose (RPG) levels more than fasting plasma glucose (FPG) levels. In a screening conducted by Harris et al., no correlation between risk factors for diabetes and the patients with hyperglycemia was found, thus recommending that all cancer patients must be screened 4–6 hours post-administration of steroids and additional monitoring may not be required if normal results are obtained on individual tests after initial dosing. Therefore, it seems challenging to determine patients that are at substantial risk for developing corticosteroid-induced hyperglycemia (C-IH) and to prevent it if typical risk factors for diabetes do not show consistency with the development of C-IH. Previously conducted studies concluded that C-IH is common in both patients with and without diabetes [odds ratio of 1.5 to 2.5 and 1.36 to 2.31 for developing glucocorticoid-induced hyperglycemia (GC-IH) in patients treated with a glucocorticoid (GC), respectively] and were strongly influenced by total GC dose, duration of use, age, and BMI (Body Mass Index) [88, 89]. Also, steroids even leading to acute elevations in blood glucose levels can have significant clinical implications demanding early identification and management in patients both with and without diabetes.

An extensive baseline examination including medical history, body weight, height, and blood pressure for all patients is recommended by Liu et al., to determine risk factors or conditions that may be influenced by corticosteroid use. Before the commencement of corticosteroid therapy, a blood glucose test should be conducted and if the initial results deviate at baseline, then home glucose monitoring is suggested [90]. The CDA recommends subsequent 48 hours monitoring for all individuals starting corticosteroid therapy and maintenance of glycemic control irrespective of the patient having pre-existing diabetes or not [91]. Interventions and continued screening may be required if the individual test results show values above the normal range (6–10 mmol/L). Therefore, it is extremely essential to monitor patients receiving corticosteroids to prevent adverse clinical implications and complications that may occur in the long term in non-palliative patients. Thorough assessment and blood-sugar-lowering medications are recommended for patients with corticosteroid-induced diabetes. Whereas patients with pre-existing diabetes may require modifying their diabetes management regimen and consideration of benefits and pitfalls before moving forward with corticosteroid therapy. Monitoring guidelines for steroid-induced diabetes recommended by the Joint British Diabetes include once-a-day monitoring for patients without diabetes and the frequency of testing should depend on the glucose level measured. Whereas diabetic patients should be tested 4 times a day. Although the guideline provides a well-structured monitoring regime, yet extensive patient education and resources to supply all patients taking steroid therapy with home capillary glucose monitoring kits are required. A study by Zanders et al. showed that adherence to glucose-lowering drug treatment declines following a cancer diagnosis [92]. Introducing different forms of medications and treatment regimens may result in overall lower effectiveness to drug treatment. To summarize, it is important to note that corticosteroids are an essential component of standard cancer treatment, but the chronic use of corticosteroids may strongly influence diabetic status and negatively affect patient outcomes. Patients prescribed corticosteroids should be closely monitored to prevent adverse effects and to effectively manage in case of their occurrence. To optimize patient care and outcomes, it is recommended that patients receive support and monitoring to prevent corticosteroid-induced diabetes and complications associated with it.

15. Neuroimaging

Dramatic outcomes are seen in clinical results of over 70% of patients receiving steroid therapy for metastatic intracranial diseases with improvement in the enhancement of the tumor, peritumoral edema, and mass effect. Computed Tomography results show a linear decrease in edema volume with measure volume of edema reduced to one-fourth times in 2 weeks of 4 mg/day steroid administration [93]. Magnetic resonance imaging shows a decrease in 10% edema volume just within a week with an average reduction in the mean volume of 4.5% within 24 hours of administering the first dose [94]. A decreased contrast enhancement with tumor is seen, suggesting partial restoration of the blood–brain barrier.

16. Drug of choice and recommendations

With the currently available evidence, dexamethasone is the most preferred drug due to its lack of mineralocorticoid activity and with its half-life being

36–54 hours provides longer duration relief from symptoms. There is currently insufficient evidence to recommend a treatment for patients with asymptomatic brain tumors without mass effect. Level 3 corticosteroids are recommended for patients with starting dose of 4–8 mg/day dexamethasone to temporarily relieve mild symptoms of increased ICP and edema related to mass effect and higher doses of 16 mg/day in divided doses, may be considered for patients with moderate to severe symptoms of increased ICP due to mass effect. A one-time trial of corticosteroid must be conducted for a duration of less than a week and results should be monitored against specific goals in particular time duration and should be discontinued if the desired results are not achieved in that duration (for example- 1 week). If the therapy is well suited and well-tolerated, it can be prescribed up to a dose of 16 mg/day (starting with minimum dose possible) for 2–3 weeks. If longer administration is required, then slow and carefully monitored tapering is required to prevent withdrawal symptoms and relapsing of initial symptoms [95–97].

17. For future investigations

Currently, there is limited information in detail about the proper use of steroids in neuro-oncology. Although a significant clinical improvement is seen in patients, an urgent need for studies addressing its dosage and toxicity exists. Future studies should focus on dosing and risk factors while limiting the side effects to potentially optimize the benefits of corticosteroid therapy.

18. Summary and discussion

Since their discovery, decades ago corticosteroids have been widely used for the treatment of brain tumors and have been considered one of the most powerful classes of tumor-induced edema reducing agents and contribute to minimizing associated neurological side effects. They are prescribed to temporarily relieve symptoms of metastatic brain tumors and only the lowest grade of recommendation can be made for mild to moderate symptoms. Higher doses may be recommended for patients with adverse symptoms tapered slowly over two weeks or longer. Sustained corticosteroid administration for long durations requires close monitoring to prevent associated immediate side effects and complications occurring in the long term. Due to well-characterized complications developing in response to steroid therapy, a need for steroid-sparing drugs such as Bevacizumab arises, but it has its limitations. Currently, there is no standard dosing regimen recommended for corticosteroids and they are prescribed depending on individual needs to maximize symptomatic relief and minimize side effects. Therefore, to bring about positive patient outcomes and to potentially optimize the benefits of corticosteroid therapy, it is suggested that future studies should focus on appropriate dosing regimens and approaches to minimize the occurrence of side effects taking into consideration the risk factors that may negatively influence the medical state.

Author details

Sunbul S. Ahmed
Independent Researcher, Delhi, India

*Address all correspondence to: sunbulahmed.neuro@outlook.com

IntechOpen

© 2021 The Author(s). Licensee IntechOpen. This chapter is distributed under the terms of the Creative Commons Attribution License (http://creativecommons.org/licenses/by/3.0), which permits unrestricted use, distribution, and reproduction in any medium, provided the original work is properly cited.

References

[1] Roth P, Happold C, Weller M. Corticosteroid use in neuro-oncology: an update. *Neurooncol Pract*. 2015;2(1):6-12. doi:10.1093/nop/npu029

[2] Streeten DH. Corticosteroid therapy. II. Complications and therapeutic indications. *JAMA*. 1975 Jun 9;232(10):1046-9. doi: 10.1001/jama.232.10.1046. PMID: 1173269.

[3] Streeten DH. Corticosteroid therapy. I. Pharmacological properties and principles of corticosteroid use. JAMA. 1975 Jun 2;232(9):944-7. doi: 10.1001/jama.232.9.944. PMID: 1173635.

[4] Ingraham FD, Matson DD, Mc Laurin RL. Cortisone and ACTH as an adjunct to the surgery of craniopharyngiomas. N. Engl. J. Med. 246(15), 568-571 (1952). • Initial study indicating usefulness of steroid in controlling and preventing postsurgical complications in brain tumors.

[5] KOFMAN S, GARVIN JS, NAGAMANI D, TAYLOR SG 3rd. Treatment of cerebral metastases from breast carcinoma with prednisolone. J Am Med Assoc. 1957 Apr 20;163(16):1473-6. doi: 10.1001/jama.1957.02970510039008. PMID: 13415910.

[6] GALICICH JH, FRENCH LA, MELBY JC. Use of dexamethasone in treatment of cerebral edema associated with brain tumors. J Lancet. 1961 Feb;81:46-53. PMID: 13703072.

[7] Bell BA. Measurement of changes in brain water in man by magnetic resonance imaging. *Ann R Coll Surg Engl*. 1989;71(6):375-380.

[8] Ryken TC, McDermott M, Robinson PD, Ammirati M, Andrews DW, Asher AL, Burri SH, Cobbs CS, Gaspar LE, Kondziolka D, Linskey ME, Loeffler JS, Mehta MP, Mikkelsen T, Olson JJ, Paleologos NA, Patchell RA, Kalkanis SN. The role of steroids in the management of brain metastases: a systematic review and evidence-based clinical practice guideline. J Neurooncol. 2010 Jan;96(1):103-14. doi: 10.1007/s11060-009-0057-4. Epub 2009 Dec 3. PMID: 19957014; PMCID: PMC2808527.

[9] Inaba H, Pui CH. Glucocorticoid use in acute lymphoblastic leukaemia. Lancet Oncol. 2010 Nov;11(11):1096-106. doi: 10.1016/S1470-2045(10)70114-5. Epub 2010 Oct 12. PMID: 20947430; PMCID: PMC3309707.

[10] al-Idrissi HY, Ibrahim EM, Abdullah KA, Ababtain WA, Boukhary HA, Macaulay HM. Antiemetic efficacy of high-dose dexamethasone: randomized, double-blind, crossover study with a combination of dexamethasone, metoclopramide and diphenhydramine. *Br J Cancer*. 1988;57(3):308-312. doi:10.1038/bjc.1988.68

[11] Todd FD 2nd, Miller CA, Yates AJ, Mervis LJ. Steroid-induced remission in primary malignant lymphoma of the central nervous system. Surg Neurol. 1986 Jul;26(1):79-84. doi: 10.1016/0090-3019(86)90068-6. PMID: 3715705.

[12] Marantidou A, Levy C, Duquesne A, Ursu R, Bailon O, Coman I, Belin C, Carpentier AF. Steroid requirements during radiotherapy for malignant gliomas. J Neurooncol. 2010 Oct;100(1):89-94. doi: 10.1007/s11060-010-0142-8. Epub 2010 Feb 26. PMID: 20186461.

[13] Shaw MM, Miller JD, Steven JL. Effect of intracranial pressure of meglumine iothalamate ventriculography. *J Neurol Neurosurg Psychiatry*. 1975;38(10):1022-1026. doi:10.1136/jnnp.38.10.1022

[14] Bracken MB, Collins WF, Freeman DF, et al. Efficacy of Methylprednisolone in Acute Spinal Cord Injury. *JAMA*. 1984;251(1):45-52. doi:10.1001/jama.1984.03340250025015

[15] Yeung TP, Yartsev S, Lee TY, et al. Relationship of computed tomography perfusion and positron emission tomography to tumour progression in malignant glioma. *J Med Radiat Sci*. 2014;61(1):4-13. doi:10.1002/jmrs.37

[16] Piette C, Munaut C, Foidart JM, Deprez M. Treating gliomas with glucocorticoids: from bedside to bench. Acta Neuropathol. 2006 Dec;112(6):651-64. doi: 10.1007/s00401-006-0100-x. Epub 2006 Jul 20. PMID: 16855833.

[17] Osawa T, Tosaka M, Nagaishi M, Yoshimoto Y. Factors affecting peritumoral brain edema in meningioma: special histological subtypes with prominently extensive edema. J Neurooncol. 2013 Jan;111(1):49-57. doi: 10.1007/s11060-012-0989-y. Epub 2012 Oct 27. PMID: 23104516.

[18] Wen PY, Schiff D, Kesari S, Drappatz J, Gigas DC, Doherty L. Medical management of patients with brain tumors. J Neurooncol. 2006 Dec;80(3):313-32. doi: 10.1007/s11060-006-9193-2. Epub 2006 Jun 29. PMID: 16807780.

[19] Papadopoulos MC, Saadoun S, Binder DK, Manley GT, Krishna S, Verkman AS. Molecular mechanisms of brain tumor edema. Neuroscience. 2004;129(4):1011-20. doi: 10.1016/j.neuroscience.2004.05.044. PMID: 15561416.

[20] Machein, M.R., Plate, K.H. VEGF in Brain Tumors. *J Neurooncol* 50, 109-120 (2000). https://doi.org/10.1023/A:1006416003964

[21] Lamszus, K., Laterra, J., Westphal, M., & Rosen, E. M. (1999). Scatter factor/hepatocyte growth factor (SF/HGF) content and function in human gliomas. *International Journal of Developmental Neuroscience*, *17*(5-6), 517-530.

[22] Wen, P.Y., Schiff, D., Kesari, S. *et al.* Medical management of patients with brain tumors. *J Neurooncol* 80, 313-332 (2006). https://doi.org/10.1007/s11060-006-9193-2

[23] Förster C, Silwedel C, Golenhofen N, Burek M, Kietz S, Mankertz J, Drenckhahn D. Occludin as direct target for glucocorticoid-induced improvement of blood-brain barrier properties in a murine in vitro system. J Physiol. 2005 Jun 1;565(Pt 2):475-86. doi: 10.1113/jphysiol.2005.084038. Epub 2005 Mar 24. PMID: 15790664; PMCID: PMC1464527.

[24] Dang TQ, Yoon N, Chasiotis H, et al. Transendothelial movement of adiponectin is restricted by glucocorticoids. *J Endocrinol*. 2017;234(2):101-114. doi:10.1530/JOE-16-0363

[25] Salvador E, Shityakov S, Förster C. Glucocorticoids and endothelial cell barrier function. Cell Tissue Res. 2014 Mar;355(3):597-605. doi: 10.1007/s00441-013-1762-z. Epub 2013 Dec 19. PMID: 24352805; PMCID: PMC3972429.

[26] Bebawy JF. Perioperative steroids for peritumoral intracranial edema: a review of mechanisms, efficacy, and side effects. J Neurosurg Anesthesiol. 2012 Jul;24(3):173-7. doi: 10.1097/ANA.0b013e3182578bb5. PMID: 22544067.

[27] Millar BM, Bezjak A, Tsao M, Sturdza A, Laperriere N. Defining the impact and contribution of steroids in patients receiving whole-brain irradiation for cerebral metastases. Clin Oncol (R Coll Radiol). 2004 Aug;16(5):339-44. doi: 10.1016/j.clon.2004.03.015. PMID: 15341437.

[28] Sionov RV, Spokoini R, Kfir-Erenfeld S, Cohen O, Yefenof E. Mechanisms regulating the susceptibility of hematopoietic malignancies to glucocorticoid-induced apoptosis. Adv Cancer Res. 2008;101:127-248. doi: 10.1016/S0065-230X(08)00406-5. PMID: 19055945.

[29] Kullmann MK, Grubbauer C, Goetsch K, Jäkel H, Podmirseg SR, Trockenbacher A, Ploner C, Cato AC, Weiss C, Kofler R, Hengst L. The p27-Skp2 axis mediates glucocorticoid-induced cell cycle arrest in T-lymphoma cells. Cell Cycle. 2013 Aug 15;12(16):2625-35. doi: 10.4161/cc.25622. Epub 2013 Jul 9. PMID: 23907123; PMCID: PMC3865052.

[30] Fan Z, Sehm T, Rauh M, Buchfelder M, Eyupoglu IY, Savaskan NE. Dexamethasone alleviates tumor-associated brain damage and angiogenesis. PLoS One. 2014 Apr 8;9(4):e93264. doi: 10.1371/journal.pone.0093264. PMID: 24714627; PMCID: PMC3979667.

[31] Langeveld CH, van Waas MP, Stoof JC, Sutanto W, de Kloet ER, Wolbers JG, Heimans JJ. Implication of glucocorticoid receptors in the stimulation of human glioma cell proliferation by dexamethasone. J Neurosci Res. 1992 Mar;31(3):524-31. doi: 10.1002/jnr.490310316. PMID: 1640503.

[32] Zibera C, Gibelli N, Butti G, Pedrazzoli P, Carbone M, Magrassi L, Robustelli della Cuna G. Proliferative effect of dexamethasone on a human glioblastoma cell line (HU 197) is mediated by glucocorticoid receptors. Anticancer Res. 1992 Sep-Oct;12(5):1571-4. PMID: 1444223.

[33] Roth P, Stupp R, Eisele G, Weller M. Treatment of primary CNS lymphoma. Curr Treat Options Neurol. 2014 Jan;16(1):277. doi: 10.1007/s11940-013-0277-y. PMID: 24343307.

[34] Grunberg SM. Antiemetic activity of corticosteroids in patients receiving cancer chemotherapy: dosing, efficacy, and tolerability analysis. Ann Oncol. 2007 Feb;18(2):233-40. doi: 10.1093/annonc/mdl347. Epub 2006 Nov 15. PMID: 17108149.

[35] Mantovani G, Macciò A, Esu S, Lai P. Evidence that cisplatin induces serotonin release from human peripheral blood mononuclear cells and that methylprednisolone inhibits this effect. Eur J Cancer. 1996 Oct;32A(11):1983-5. doi: 10.1016/0959-8049(96)00204-3. PMID: 8943685.

[36] Suzuki T, Sugimoto M, Koyama H, Mashimo T, Uchida I. Inhibitory effect of glucocorticoids on human-cloned 5-hydroxytryptamine3A receptor expressed in xenopus oocytes. Anesthesiology. 2004 Sep;101(3):660-5. doi: 10.1097/00000542-200409000-00014. PMID: 15329590.

[37] Hempen C, Weiss E, Hess CF. Dexamethasone treatment in patients with brain metastases and primary brain tumors: do the benefits outweigh the side-effects? Support Care Cancer. 2002 May;10(4):322-8. doi: 10.1007/s00520-001-0333-0. Epub 2002 Feb 9. PMID: 12029432.

[38] Vecht CJ, Hovestadt A, Verbiest HB, van Vliet JJ, van Putten WL. Dose-effect relationship of dexamethasone on Karnofsky performance in metastatic brain tumors: a randomized study of doses of 4, 8, and 16 mg per day. Neurology. 1994 Apr;44(4):675-80. doi: 10.1212/wnl.44.4.675. PMID: 8164824.

[39] Weissman DE, Janjan NA, Erickson B, Wilson FJ, Greenberg M, Ritch PS, Anderson T, Hansen RM, Chitambar CR, Lawton CA, et al. Twice-daily tapering dexamethasone treatment during cranial radiation for newly diagnosed brain metastases. J Neurooncol. 1991 Dec;11(3):235-9. doi: 10.1007/BF00165531. PMID: 1726656.

[40] Oki K, Yamane K. Therapies for adrenal insufficiency. Expert Opin Pharmacother. 2007 Jun;8(9):1283-91. doi: 10.1517/14656566.8.9.1283. PMID: 17563263.

[41] Koehler PJ. Use of corticosteroids in neuro-oncology. Anticancer Drugs. 1995 Feb;6(1):19-33. doi: 10.1097/00001813-199502000-00002. PMID: 7756680.

[42] Grossman E, Messerli FH. Drug-induced hypertension: an unappreciated cause of secondary hypertension. Am J Med. 2012 Jan;125(1):14-22. doi: 10.1016/j.amjmed.2011.05.024. PMID: 22195528.

[43] Conn HO, Blitzer BL. Nonassociation of adrenocorticosteroid therapy and peptic ulcer. N Engl J Med. 1976 Feb 26;294(9):473-9. doi: 10.1056/NEJM197602262940905. PMID: 173997.

[44] Strom BL, Carson JL, Schinnar R, et al. Upper gastrointestinal tract bleeding from oral potassium chloride. Comparative risk from micro-encapsulated vs wax-matrix formulations. Archives of Internal Medicine. 1987 May;147(5):954-957. DOI: 10.1001/archinte.1987.00370050146025. PMID: 3495244.

[45] Conn HO, Poynard T. Adrenocorticosteroid administration and peptic ulcer: a critical analysis. J Chronic Dis. 1985;38(6):457-68. doi: 10.1016/0021-9681(85)90028-1. PMID: 3891768.

[46] Steinbuch M, Youket TE, Cohen S. Oral glucocorticoid use is associated with an increased risk of fracture. Osteoporos Int. 2004 Apr;15(4):323-8. doi: 10.1007/s00198-003-1548-3. Epub 2004 Feb 5. PMID: 14762652.

[47] Kanis JA, Johansson H, Oden A, Johnell O, de Laet C, Melton III LJ, Tenenhouse A, Reeve J, Silman AJ, Pols HA, Eisman JA, McCloskey EV, Mellstrom D. A meta-analysis of prior corticosteroid use and fracture risk. J Bone Miner Res. 2004 Jun;19(6):893-9. doi: 10.1359/JBMR.040134. Epub 2004 Jan 27. PMID: 15125788.

[48] Grossman JM, Gordon R, Ranganath VK, Deal C, Caplan L, Chen W, Curtis JR, Furst DE, McMahon M, Patkar NM, Volkmann E, Saag KG. American College of Rheumatology 2010 recommendations for the prevention and treatment of glucocorticoid-induced osteoporosis. Arthritis Care Res (Hoboken). 2010 Nov;62(11):1515-26. doi: 10.1002/acr.20295. Epub 2010 Jul 26. Erratum in: Arthritis Care Res (Hoboken). 2012 Mar;64(3):464. PMID: 20662044.

[49] Farhat G, Yamout B, Mikati MA, Demirjian S, Sawaya R, El-Hajj Fuleihan G. Effect of antiepileptic drugs on bone density in ambulatory patients. Neurology. 2002 May 14;58(9):1348-53. doi: 10.1212/wnl.58.9.1348. PMID: 12011279.

[50] Feldkamp J, Becker A, Witte OW, Scharff D, Scherbaum WA. Long-term anticonvulsant therapy leads to low bone mineral density--evidence for direct drug effects of phenytoin and carbamazepine on human osteoblast-like cells. Exp Clin Endocrinol Diabetes. 2000;108(1):37-43. doi: 10.1055/s-0032-1329213. PMID: 10768830.

[51] Shen C, Chen F, Zhang Y, Guo Y, Ding M. Association between use of antiepileptic drugs and fracture risk: a systematic review and meta-analysis. Bone. 2014 Jul;64:246-53. doi: 10.1016/j.bone.2014.04.018. Epub 2014 Apr 26. PMID: 24780876.

[52] Lipton A. New therapeutic agents for the treatment of bone diseases. Expert Opin Biol Ther. 2005 Jun;5(6):817-32. doi: 10.1517/14712598.5.6.817. PMID: 15952912.

[53] Streeten DH. Corticosteroid therapy. II. Complications and therapeutic indications. JAMA. 1975 Jun;232(10):1046-1049. DOI: 10.1001/jama.232.10.1046. PMID: 1173269.

[54] Lewis DA, Smith RE. Steroid-induced psychiatric syndromes. A report of 14 cases and a review of the literature. J Affect Disord. 1983 Nov;5(4):319-32. doi: 10.1016/0165-0327(83)90022-8. PMID: 6319464.

[55] Bolanos SH, Khan DA, Hanczyc M, Bauer MS, Dhanani N, Brown ES. Assessment of mood states in patients receiving long-term corticosteroid therapy and in controls with patient-rated and clinician-rated scales. Ann Allergy Asthma Immunol. 2004 May;92(5):500-5. doi: 10.1016/S1081-1206(10)61756-5. PMID: 15191017.

[56] Brown ES, Suppes T, Khan DA, Carmody TJ 3rd. Mood changes during prednisone bursts in outpatients with asthma. J Clin Psychopharmacol. 2002 Feb;22(1):55-61. doi: 10.1097/00004714-200202000-00009. PMID: 11799343.

[57] Sonino N, Fava GA, Raffi AR, Boscaro M, Fallo F. Clinical correlates of major depression in Cushing's disease. Psychopathology. 1998 Nov-Dec;31(6):302-6. doi: 10.1159/000029054. PMID: 9780396.

[58] Qian T, Guo X, Levi AD, Vanni S, Shebert RT, Sipski ML. High-dose methylprednisolone may cause myopathy in acute spinal cord injury patients. Spinal Cord. 2005 Apr;43(4):199-203. doi: 10.1038/sj.sc.3101681. PMID: 15534623.

[59] Steinberg KP, Hudson LD, Goodman RB, Hough CL, Lanken PN, Hyzy R, Thompson BT, Ancukiewicz M; National Heart, Lung, and Blood Institute Acute Respiratory Distress Syndrome (ARDS) Clinical Trials Network. Efficacy and safety of corticosteroids for persistent acute respiratory distress syndrome. N Engl J Med. 2006 Apr 20;354(16):1671-84. doi: 10.1056/NEJMoa051693. PMID: 16625008

[60] Dekhuijzen PN, Decramer M. Steroid-induced myopathy and its significance to respiratory disease: a known disease rediscovered. Eur Respir J. 1992 Sep;5(8):997-1003. PMID: 1426209.

[61] Kimura K, Kanda F, Okuda S, Chihara K. Insulin-like growth factor 1 inhibits glucocorticoid-induced glutamine synthetase activity in cultured L6 rat skeletal muscle cells. Neurosci Lett. 2001 Apr 20;302(2-3):154-6. doi: 10.1016/s0304-3940(01)01667-6. PMID: 11290410.

[62] Dietrich J, Rao K, Pastorino S, Kesari S. Corticosteroids in brain cancer patients: benefits and pitfalls. Expert Review of Clinical Pharmacology. 2011 Mar;4(2):233-242. DOI: 10.1586/ecp.11.1. PMID: 21666852; PMCID: PMC3109638.

[63] Frieze DA. Musculoskeletal pain associated with corticosteroid therapy in cancer. Curr Pain Headache Rep. 2010 Aug;14(4):256-60. doi: 10.1007/s11916-010-0120-z. PMID: 20490741.

[64] Arnaldo Neves Da Silva, David Schiff. Adrenal insufficiency secondary to glucocorticoid withdrawal in patients with brain tumor, Surgical Neurology, Volume 67, Issue 5,2007,Pages 508-510, ISSN 0090-3019 https://doi.org/10.1016/j.surneu.2006.07.018.

[65] Lansang MC, Hustak LK. Glucocorticoid-induced diabetes and adrenal suppression: how to detect and manage them. Cleve Clin J Med. 2011 Nov;78(11):748-56. doi: 10.3949/ccjm.78a.10180. PMID: 22049542.

[66] Henson JW, Jalaj JK, Walker RW, Stover DE, Fels AO. Pneumocystis carinii pneumonia in patients with

primary brain tumors. Arch Neurol. 1991 Apr;48(4):406-9. doi: 10.1001/archneur.1991.00530160074017. PMID: 2012515.

[67] Maria Grazia Cifone, Graziella Migliorati, Raffaella Parroni, Cristina Marchetti, Danilo Millimaggi, Angela Santoni, Carlo Riccardi; Dexamethasone-Induced Thymocyte Apoptosis: Apoptotic Signal Involves the Sequential Activation of Phosphoinositide-Specific Phospholipase C, Acidic Sphingomyelinase, and Caspases. *Blood* 1999; 93 (7): 2282-2296. doi: https://doi.org/10.1182/blood.V93.7.2282

[68] Herold, M.J., McPherson, K.G. & Reichardt, H.M. Glucocorticoids in T cell apoptosis and function. *Cell. Mol. Life Sci.* 63, 60 (2006). https://doi.org/10.1007/s00018-005-5390-y

[69] Franchimont, D., Galon, J., Gadina, M., Visconti, R., Zhou, Y. J., Aringer, M., ... & O'Shea, J. J. (2000). Inhibition of Th1 immune response by glucocorticoids: dexamethasone selectively inhibits IL-12-induced Stat4 phosphorylation in T lymphocytes. *The Journal of Immunology*, 164(4), 1768-1774.

[70] Baschant, U., & Tuckermann, J. (2010). The role of the glucocorticoid receptor in inflammation and immunity. *The Journal of steroid biochemistry and molecular biology*, 120(2-3), 69-75.

[71] Callahan MK, Wolchok JD. At the bedside: CTLA-4- and PD-1-blocking antibodies in cancer immunotherapy. J Leukoc Biol. 2013 Jul;94(1):41-53. doi: 10.1189/jlb.1212631. Epub 2013 May 10. PMID: 23667165; PMCID: PMC4051187.

[72] Sampson, J. H., Vlahovic, G., Desjardins, A., Friedman, H. S., Baehring, J. M., Hafler, D., ... & Reardon, D. A. (2014). Randomized phase IIb study of nivolumab (anti-PD-1; BMS-936558, ONO-4538) alone or in combination with ipilimumab versus bevacizumab in patients (pts) with recurrent glioblastoma (GBM).

[73] Chalk JB, Ridgeway K, Brophy T, Yelland JD, Eadie MJ. Phenytoin impairs the bioavailability of dexamethasone in neurological and neurosurgical patients. J Neurol Neurosurg Psychiatry. 1984 Oct;47(10):1087-90. doi: 10.1136/jnnp.47.10.1087. PMID: 6502166; PMCID: PMC1028038.

[74] Choi Y, Thrasher K, Werk EE Jr, Sholiton LJ, Olinger C. Effect of diphenylhydantoin on cortisol kinetics in humans. J Pharmacol Exp Ther. 1971 Jan;176(1):27-34. PMID: 4936459.

[75] Brooks SM, Werk EE, Ackerman SJ, Sullivan I, Thrasher K. Adverse effects of phenobarbital on corticosteroid metabolism in patients with bronchial asthma. The New England Journal of Medicine. 1972 May;286(21):1125-1128. DOI: 10.1056/nejm197205252862103. PMID: 4553339.

[76] Lawson LA, Blouin RA, Smith RB, Rapp RP, Young AB. Phenytoin-dexamethasone interaction: a previously unreported observation. Surgical Neurology. 1981 Jul;16(1):23-24. DOI: 10.1016/s0090-3019(81)80054-7. PMID: 7280966.

[77] Robert L. Ruff, Joseph Weissmann, Endocrine Myopathies, Neurologic Clinics, Volume 6, Issue 3,1988, Pages 575-592, ISSN 0733-8619, https://doi.org/10.1016/S0733-8619(18)30862-4.

[78] Asconapé JJ, Penry JK. Use of antiepileptic drugs in the presence of liver and kidney diseases: a review. Epilepsia. 1982 ;23 Suppl 1:S65-79. DOI: 10.1111/j.1528-1157.1982.tb06092.x. PMID: 6814902.

[79] Das A, Banik NL, Patel SJ, Ray SK. Dexamethasone protected human glioblastoma U87MG cells from temozolomide induced apoptosis by

maintaining Bax:Bcl-2 ratio and preventinDas A, Banik NL, Patel SJ, Ray SK. Dexamethasone protected human glioblastoma U87MG cells from temozolomide induced apoptosis by maintaining Bax:Bcl-2 ratio and preventing proteolytic activities. *Mol Cancer*. 2004;3(1):36. Published 2004 Dec 8. doi:10.1186/1476-4598-3-36g proteolytic activities. *Mol Cancer*. 2004;3(1):36. Published 2004 Dec 8. doi:10.1186/1476-4598-3-36

[80] Tjuvajev J, Uehara H, Desai R, Beattie B, Matei C, Zhou Y, Kreek MJ, Koutcher J, Blasberg R. Corticotropin-releasing factor decreases vasogenic brain edema. Cancer Res. 1996 Mar 15;56(6):1352-60. PMID: 8640825.

[81] Dietrich J, Rao K, Pastorino S, Kesari S. Corticosteroids in brain cancer patients: benefits and pitfalls. Expert Review of Clinical Pharmacology. 2011 Mar;4(2):233-242. DOI: 10.1586/ecp.11.1. PMID: 21666852; PMCID: PMC3109638.

[82] Gerstner ER, Duda DG, di Tomaso E, Ryg PA, Loeffler JS, Sorensen AG, Ivy P, Jain RK, Batchelor TT. VEGF inhibitors in the treatment of cerebral edema in patients with brain cancer. Nat Rev Clin Oncol. 2009 Apr;6(4):229-36. doi: 10.1038/nrclinonc.2009.14. PMID: 19333229; PMCID: PMC4793889.

[83] Tjuvajev J, Uehara H, Desai R, Beattie B, Matei C, Zhou Y, Kreek MJ, Koutcher J, Blasberg R. Corticotropin-releasing factor decreases vasogenic brain edema. Cancer Res. 1996 Mar 15;56(6):1352-60. PMID: 8640825.

[84] Villalona-Calero MA, Eckardt J, Burris H, Kraynak M, Fields-Jones S, Bazan C, Lancaster J, Hander T, Goldblum R, Hammond L, Bari A, Drengler R, Rothenberg M, Hadovsky G, Von Hoff DD. A phase I trial of human corticotropin-releasing factor (hCRF) in patients with peritumoral brain edema. Ann Oncol. 1998 Jan;9(1):71-7. doi: 10.1023/a:1008251426425. PMID: 9541686.

[85] Recht L, Mechtler LL, Wong ET, O'Connor PC, Rodda BE. Steroid-sparing effect of corticorelin acetate in peritumoral cerebral edema is associated with improvement in steroid-induced myopathy. J Clin Oncol. 2013 Mar 20;31(9):1182-7. doi: 10.1200/JCO.2012.43.9455. Epub 2013 Feb 4. PMID: 23382470.

[86] Nathoo N, Barnett GH, Golubic M, The eicosanoid cascade: possible role in gliomas and meningiomas, *Journal of Clinical Pathology* 2004;57:6-13.

[87] Portnow J, Suleman S, Grossman SA, Eller S, Carson K. A cyclooxygenase-2 (COX-2) inhibitor compared with dexamethasone in a survival study of rats with intracerebral 9L gliosarcomas. Neuro-oncology. 2002 Jan;4(1):22-25. DOI: 10.1093/neuonc/4.1.22. PMID: 11772429; PMCID: PMC1920630.

[88] Clore JN, Thurby-Hay L. Glucocorticoid-induced hyperglycemia. Endocr Pract. 2009 Jul-Aug;15(5):469-74. doi: 10.4158/EP08331.RAR. PMID: 19454391.

[89] Kwon S, Hermayer KL, Hermayer K. Glucocorticoid-induced hyperglycemia. Am J Med Sci. 2013 Apr;345(4):274-277. doi: 10.1097/MAJ.0b013e31828a6a01. PMID: 23531958.

[90] Liu D, Ahmet A, Ward L, Krishnamoorthy P, Mandelcorn ED, Leigh R, Brown JP, Cohen A, Kim H. A practical guide to the monitoring and management of the complications of systemic corticosteroid therapy. Allergy Asthma Clin Immunol. 2013 Aug 15;9(1):30. doi: 10.1186/1710-1492-9-30. PMID: 23947590; PMCID: PMC3765115.

[91] Canadian Diabetes Association Clinical Practice Guidelines Expert

Committee, Cheng AY. Canadian Diabetes Association 2013 clinical practice guidelines for the prevention and management of diabetes in Canada. Introduction. Can J Diabetes. 2013 Apr;37 Suppl 1:S1-3. doi: 10.1016/j.jcjd.2013.01.009. Epub 2013 Mar 26. PMID: 24070926.

[92] Zanders, M.M.J., Haak, H.R., van Herk-Sukel, M.P.P. et al. Impact of cancer on use of glucose-lowering drug treatment in individuals with diabetes: potential mechanisms. Reply to Pouwer F [letter]. *Diabetologia* 58, 1380-1381 (2015). https://doi.org/10.1007/s00125-015-3578-8

[93] Andersen C, Astrup J, Gyldensted C. Quantitation of peritumoural oedema and the effect of steroids using NMR-relaxation time imaging and blood-brain barrier analysis. Acta Neurochir Suppl (Wien). 1994;60:413-5. doi: 10.1007/978-3-7091-9334-1_112. PMID: 7976605.

[94] Hatam A, Yu ZY, Bergström M, Berggren BM, Greitz T. Effect of dexamethasone treatment on peritumoral brain edema: evaluation by computed tomography. J Comput Assist Tomogr. 1982 Jun;6(3):586-92. doi: 10.1097/00004728-198206000-00025. PMID: 6284815.

[95] Soffietti R, Cornu P, Delattre JY, Grant R, Graus F, Grisold W, Heimans J, Hildebrand J, Hoskin P, Kalljo M, Krauseneck P, Marosi C, Siegal T, Vecht C. EFNS Guidelines on diagnosis and treatment of brain metastases: report of an EFNS Task Force. Eur J Neurol. 2006 Jul;13(7):674-81. doi: 10.1111/j.1468-1331.2006.01506.x. PMID: 16834697.

[96] Gaspar LE, Gutin PH, Rogers L, Schneider JF, Larson D, Bloomer WD, Buckley JA, Gibbs FA, Lewin AA, Loeffler JS, Malcolm AW, Mendenhall WM, Schupak KD, Shaw EG, Simpson JR, Wharam MD Jr,
Leibel S. Pre-irradiation evaluation and management of brain metastases. American College of Radiology. ACR Appropriateness Criteria. Radiology. 2000 Jun;215 Suppl:1105-10. PMID: 11037534.

[97] Millar, B. M., Bezjak, A., Tsao, M., Sturdza, A., & Laperriere, N. (2004). Defining the impact and contribution of steroids in patients receiving whole-brain irradiation for cerebral metastases. *Clinical Oncology*, 16(5), 339-344.

Chapter 6

Corticosteroid Replacement Therapy

Michael C. Onyema

Abstract

The advent of synthetic corticosteroids in the 20th century provided a vital breakthrough in the management of adrenal insufficiency. In this chapter we review the main indications and guidance for appropriate hormone replacement and also look into the management of therapy during special circumstances. For decades hydrocortisone has remained the cornerstone for glucocorticoid replacement but we explore the alternatives including recently introduced modified-release drug preparations and the future treatment considerations currently undergoing research and pre-clinical trials.

Keywords: Corticosteroids, Glucocorticoids, Hormone Replacement, Adrenal Crisis, Sick Day Rules, Novel Therapies

1. Introduction

Corticosteroid replacement therapy in adrenal insufficiency namely glucocorticoids such as hydrocortisone serve as life sustaining therapy therefore its appropriate administration when stable or unwell is of vital importance. In this chapter we explore the indications and guidance for corticosteroid replacement therapies including management during special circumstances such as emergencies, pregnancy and breastfeeding. We also look at current novel therapies and look towards future perspectives on treatment therapies under research.

2. Overview

Adrenal insufficiency was first postulated by the physician Thomas Addison of Guy's Hospital London in 1855. He characterized the condition of progressive anemia, bronze skin pigmentation and low blood pressure in disease of the 'suprarenal capsules' – now known as Addison's disease [1]. This is a condition epitomized by insufficient production of steroid hormones from the adrenal cortex: primarily glucocorticoids from the zona fasiculata but can also affect mineralocorticoid and adrenal androgen production (from the zona glomerulosa and zona reticularis respectively).

It has historically carried a high mortality rate until the advent of therapeutic corticosteroid preparations in the mid-20th century. Life expectancy is generally considered normal with the application of appropriate replacement therapy but there is a growing body of evidence of highlighting increased morbidity and reduced life expectancy likely related to increased cardiovascular risk with hormonal over replacement and adrenal crises. Glucocorticoid administration is essentially life sustaining therapy; some patients will also require the co-administration of mineralocorticoids drugs and the adrenal androgen *dehydroepiandrosterone* (DHEA). The importance of replacement therapy is not only to starve off symptoms of hormone deficiency (including fatigue, muscle weakness, dizziness, weight loss, low mood, low libido) but also is imperative in maintaining key physiological processes (including gluconeogenesis, immune modulation, electrolyte balance, metabolism and haemodynamic modulation).

3. Conditions necessitating hormone replacement

Adrenal insufficiency requiring corticosteroid hormone replacement therapy is triggered by conditions or factors interrupting the normal function of the hypothalamic–pituitary–adrenal axis (HPA axis). Most causes are acquired in nature rather than congenital and can be divided into *primary adrenal insufficiency* (direct adrenal hormone synthesis dysfunction) and *secondary adrenal insufficiency* (inadequate ACTH production).

Hormone deficiency is a deficit deemed unable to meet the physiological demands of the body, most notably in response to stress. In deficiency states glucocorticoid replacement therapy is always required. However because mineralocorticoid and adrenal androgen production is only partially mediated by ACTH; replacement therapy of these hormones is not usually required in secondary adrenal insufficiency.

The most common cause of primary adrenal insufficiency in the developed world is autoimmune in nature – approximately 70% of cases [2] with antibodies present against the 21-hydroxylase enzyme.

Other notable causes of primary adrenal insufficiency include:

- Infection (e.g. tuberculosis)

- Malignancy (e.g. adrenal metastases)

- Iatrogenic (e.g. post-adrenalectomy, ketoconazole)

- Inherited (e.g. congenital adrenal hyperplasia).

Notable causes of secondary adrenal insufficiency include:

- Pituitary tumors

- Hypothalamic/pituitary infections or inflammation (e.g. tuberculosis, lymphocytic hypophysititis)

- Iatrogenic (e.g. post transpenoidal surgery, radiotherapy)

- Isolated ACTH deficiency

- Long term exogenous glucocorticoid therapy (causing suppression of HPA axis).

Corticosteroid replacement therapy is often required lifelong but, depending on the cause, therapy may be able to be safely withdrawn in future if adrenal function recovers.

4. Historical perspective

Early animal studies in 1930 proved bovine adrenal extracts could transiently treat symptoms of adrenal insufficiency. The later production of synthetic desoxycorticosterone acetate in 1938 was the major step in providing a therapeutic agent to successfully treat adrenal insufficiency. In 1950 commercial therapeutic use of hydrocortisone was established after recognition of cortisol as the key end product of adrenal cortex hormone synthesis [3]. To current day hydrocortisone therapy still remains the mainstay replacement therapeutic drug.

5. Assessing for glucocorticoid deficiency

Suspicion of glucocorticoid deficiency can be initially indicated by typical symptomology, hypotension and skin hyperpigmentation (in cases of primary adrenal insufficiency associated with excess ACTH production). Baseline biochemistry can often reveal a combination of hyponatraemia, hyperkalaemia or hypoglycaemia. Morning cortisol and ACTH levels are useful markers in preliminary testing with cortisol levels <140 nmol/L being indicative of deficiency. Elevated or low ACTH levels assist in defining primary vs. secondary adrenal insufficiency respectively (an ACTH level two-fold the upper reference range is consistent with primary adrenal insufficiency). There is no evidence to support the role of random cortisol levels to diagnose adrenal insufficiency [4].

A corticotropin (ACTH) stimulation test is considered the gold standard confirmatory test in primary adrenal insufficiency. Typically baseline cortisol and ACTH levels are taken followed by the administration of a 250 μg IV corticotropin bolus and further monitoring of cortisol levels at 30 minutes and/or 60 minutes. Acceptable cortisol levels indicating sufficient adrenal response remain controversial. Newer monoclonal antibody cortisol immunoassays (including Roche II Elecsys) display increased sensitivities and specificity, allowing for a diagnostic peak cortisol threshold of >400 nmol/L [5].

In cases of secondary adrenal insufficiency an insulin tolerance test – ITT (or insulin stress test) has proved to be more successful in detecting cortisol deficiency in comparison to corticotropin stimulation testing in studies [6]. In testing the aim is to induce extreme hypoglycaemia (<2.2 mmol/L) with the administration of (0.15 units/kg soluble insulin). In normal circumstances hypoglycaemia leads to hypersecretion of the insulin antagonizing hormones ACTH and growth hormone (GH) from the anterior pituitary gland; with a subsequent cortisol rise of <500 nmol/L is considered an inadequate response. It is a potentially harmful test and therefore should be undertaken with care. It is contraindicated in ischaemic heart disease, epilepsy and severe panhypopituitarism; in these circumstances glucagon is often used instead of insulin as the stress provocation agent. Notable scenarios for effective ITT utility include following borderline corticotropin stimulation testing and following recent pituitary surgery [7].

6. Glucocorticoid replacement

Human endogenous glucocorticoid release follows a circadian rhythm i.e. an internal process following a 24 hour cycle. There are also 60–90 minute ultradian oscillations during the day to consider. These processes are ultimately under the control of the hypothalamic suprachiasmatic nuclei (SCN) and subsequent corticotropin-releasing hormone (CRH) secretion that stimulates pituitary ACTH synthesis variably [8]. The circadian rhythm may be altered by changes to activity, aging, sleep and mood.

Typically in a 24 hour profile we see an early morning ACTH/cortisol peak with declining levels during the daytime until quiescence at midnight. There is then a brisk elevation during late sleep leading on to the early morning peak we see at the beginning of the cycle. It is this pattern that administered glucocorticoid therapy ideally attempts to recreate.

Hydrocortisone is the most commonly administered glucocorticoid therapeutic agent for adrenal insufficiency. Clinic data from the UK revealed 72% of patients were managed with hydrocortisone, 26% with prednisolone and 2% with modified release hydrocortisone [9]. Data from the European Adrenal Insufficiency Registry.

(EU-AIR) study additionally showed that over 80% of patients were on conventional hydrocortisone replacement therapy on enrolment [10].

In clinical practice the use of hydrocortisone or prednisolone are often preferable due to their more predictable pharmacokinetics compared to their precursor hormones cortisone and prednisone [9]. The normal functioning adrenal glands are thought to produce 5-10 mg cortisol per m^2 body surface area/per day; this equates to an oral hydrocortisone dose of 15-25 mg/per day for an adult [11]. Due to its short half-life hydrocortisone is usually given in 2–3 divided doses with the largest dose in the morning and the last dose at least 4–6 hours prior to bedtime to avoid sleep disturbances. Prednisolone is a glucocorticoid analogue with a greater avidity for the glucocorticoid (GC) receptor. Studies have shown once daily prednisolone administration to be superior to thrice-daily hydrocortisone in imitating the physiological cortisol profile and reducing over replacement at a recommended dose of 3-5 mg daily [12]. Other potential benefits of prednisolone include cost-effectiveness and increased medication compliance although the comparative long-term metabolic side effect risk between hydrocortisone and once daily prednisolone remain controversial [13–15].

6.1 Novel glucocorticoid replacement therapies

Plenadren® is a novel modified-release form of hydrocortisone given European marketing authorization in November 2011. This once daily preparation contains both immediate-release and extended-release components with an aim to more closely mimic the body's physiological circadian rhythm. It can be considered an alternative for patients who continue to feel unwell on conventional therapy, given typically at a dose of 15-25 mg daily. Evidence from 2 randomized-controlled trials (RCTs) has shown a reduction in CV disease risk parameters with modified release hydrocortisone compared to conventional therapy [9]. Though Plenadren® carries a significantly higher cost basis to the other traditional therapeutic glucocorticoid medications and carries a higher vulnerability to malabsorption during intercurrent gastrointestinal illness [16].

Chronocort® is another novel modified-release form of hydrocortisone with delayed absorption, taken at night with an aim to replicate the physiological early morning cortisol rise and circadian rhythm more closely. It has completed phase III trials for the use in adrenal insufficiency and congenital adrenal hyperplasia; currently awaiting licensing authorization in Europe.

Continuous subcutaneous hydrocortisone infusions (CSHI) were first used from 2007. These offer variable hydrocortisone delivery often through traditional 'insulin pumps' helping to replicate the circadian rhythm most accurately compared to oral therapies. This requires a high degree of patient education and autonomy. Those that can benefit include those patients poorly tolerant or responsive to tablets especially in light of gastric absorption issues. Studies using continuous infusions have shown better normalization of morning ACTH levels [3]. From minimal comparative studies there has been no consistent evidence of improvement in subjective health outcomes. One RCT showed a mild increase in weight and fasting glucose levels in patients on hydrocortisone infusions but it was felt likely attributable to supra-physiological hydrocortisone dosing (based on elevated urinary and salivary cortisol levels in comparison to the oral hydrocortisone group recipients).

The therapy remains uncommon in healthcare systems, potentially cumbersome and is best commenced by experienced endocrine units. The Endocrine Society 2016 guidance on management of primary adrenal insufficiency suggests reserving such treatment for patients encountering major difficulties on conventional therapy [4].

6.2 Mineralocorticoid replacement

Most patients with primary adrenal insufficiency will exhibit mineralocorticoid deficiency. As release is also under the control of the renin-angiotensin system (RAS) deficiencies can also be caused by reduced renin levels (*hyporeninemic hypoaldosteronism*) due to conditions including diabetic nephropathy, sickle cell anemia, myeloma and medications (e.g. NSAID, beta blockers, Ciclosporin).

Mineralocorticoids are important in circulatory homeostasis and salt balance. Deficiencies can lead to salt craving, postural hypotension, dizziness, hyponatraemia, hyperkalaemia and reduced cognition. To alleviate symptoms replacement therapy is typically met through the use of fludrocortisone and as well advice to increase dietary salt. The Endocrine Society 2016 guidance on management of primary adrenal insufficiency suggests a starting dose of fludrocortisone 50-100mcg in those with confirmed deficiency (assessed by way of plasma renin and aldosterone levels) [4]. Typically higher doses of replacement therapy are required for the more physically active and less sedentary patient cohorts [11].

6.3 Androgen replacement

Primary adrenal insufficiency can also affect adrenal androgen reserve. In women adrenal androgen precursors DHEA and androstenedione are major contributors to the physiological production of potent androgens and oestogen in the zona reticularis. Clinically deficiencies can lead to notable axillary and pubic hair loss.

The benefits of replacement therapy are not very clear. There is some evidence to suggest that health related quality of life markers can be improved with synthetic DHEA in patients with primary adrenal insufficiency [3]. The Endocrine Society notes that there is insufficient evidence to advocate routine androgen replacement therapy but suggests a 6 month trial of DHEA for women with ongoing symptoms of low libido, low mood and/or low energy levels despite optimized glucocorticoid and mineralocorticoid replacement. A single DHEA dose of 25-50 mg in the morning can be considered in the first instance [4].

7. Glucocorticoids *(dose titration and monitoring)*

Signs of glucocorticoid under replacement may include development of lethargy, nausea, headaches, muscle aches, weight loss, increased skin pigmentation and hypotension. Biochemistry may reveal elevated potassium levels and reduced sodium levels. On the contrary signs of over replacement may include weight gain, facial puffiness, insomnia, and glucose intolerance. Longer term over replacement can lead to established hypertension, type 2 diabetes mellitus, osteoporosis and increased overall CV risk. Stability of replacement therapy is therefore of importance to achieve and optimal dosing will vary between individuals with differences including body composition, absorption, metabolism and protein binding.

The Endocrine Society recommends measuring the adequacy of replacement primarily with clinical assessment including weight, postural blood pressure, energy levels and signs of frank glucocorticoid excess. It is advised against routine hormonal monitoring, instead for titration of treatment based on clinical response. In cases where malabsorption is suspected further analysis with serum or salivary cortisol day curves are recommended as a guide for dosing [4] but there is a lack of reliable biomarkers for treatment monitoring and notably measured concentrations of ACTH are not a useful parameter [11, 17].

7.1 Mineralocorticoids *(dose titration and monitoring)*

Fludrocortisone under replacement is common and can be often seen compensated by supra-physiological glucocorticoid doses which puts patients at high risk for developing the subsequent metabolic sequelae associated with hypercortisolaemia. Signs of over replacement with fludrocortisone include hypertension and oedema. The Endocrine Society recommends reviewing replacement dosing clinically by assessing for salt craving, postural hypotension, oedema and blood electrolytes (aiming for normokalaemia). It is also advised the hypertension is initially managed by dose reduction following the addition of antihypertensive agents if necessary [4].

It is common to use plasma renin activity as a guide for appropriate Fludrocortisone replacement although the data to support its usefulness is limited. The ideal renin target levels lie in the upper reference range. Caution must be taken with interpretation as levels can be affected by variables such as body position, time of day and medications. Additionally liquorice and grapefruit potentiate the mineralocorticoid effects of hydrocortisone and should thus be avoided [4, 11].

7.2 Androgens *(dose titration and monitoring)*

Adequate replacement with DHEA may be noted by improved libido, mood and energy levels on assessment. The Endocrine Society recommends taking morning (pre-dose) DHEAS levels to guide treatment, aiming for levels in the mid-normal range [4]. Levels may be taken by saliva, serum or urine. There are however potential side effects of DHEA therapy related to androgen excess including hirsutism, acne, deepened voice and hair loss. Studies have shown some benefits to bone density, lean mass and psychological wellbeing scores [18].

8. Sick day rules, emergency advice and adrenal crises management

During periods of acute illness and physiological stress there are increased demands of cortisol production placed on the body. Glucocorticoid doses must be increased accordingly to match demands and prevent the onset of an adrenal crisis (commonly evidenced by hypotension, nausea, abdominal pain, reduced consciousness and electrolytes disturbances). Therefore in the presence of illness such as infection with fever, diarrhea/vomiting, significant trauma or significant psychological stress/bereavement; there is general consensus that glucocorticoid doses should be doubled for the duration of illness/antibiotic course (patients taking Plenadren® are best placed switching to hydrocortisone during these periods for better physiological cortisol profiling). Management of therapy is also of important consideration in the perioperative setting with general advice of giving hydrocortisone 100 mg IV or IM just prior to surgery or at anesthetic induction and weaning doses back to baseline during the recovery period as applicable. Fludrocortisone doses do not need to be routinely increased as hydrocortisone/prednisolone also convey mineralocorticoid receptor activity which is potentiated at higher doses due to saturation of 11β-hydroxysteroid dehydrogenase enzyme (this is not the case for dexamethasone which does not exert mineralocorticoid activity).

At diagnosis patients should be well educated in the sick day management of steroid therapy often provided through endocrine specialist nurses and reinforced

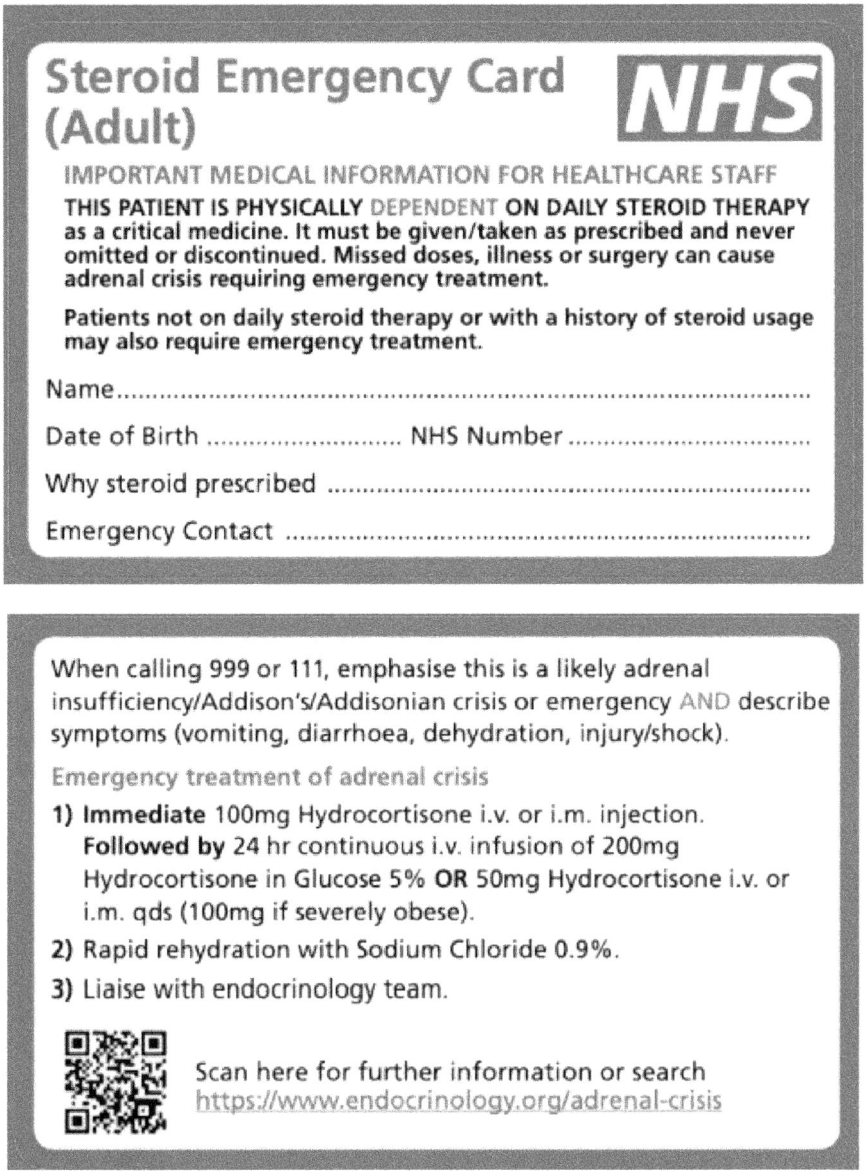

Steroid Emergency Card (Adult)

NHS

IMPORTANT MEDICAL INFORMATION FOR HEALTHCARE STAFF

THIS PATIENT IS PHYSICALLY DEPENDENT ON DAILY STEROID THERAPY as a critical medicine. It must be given/taken as prescribed and never omitted or discontinued. Missed doses, illness or surgery can cause adrenal crisis requiring emergency treatment.

Patients not on daily steroid therapy or with a history of steroid usage may also require emergency treatment.

Name ....

Date of Birth .... NHS Number ....

Why steroid prescribed ....

Emergency Contact ....

When calling 999 or 111, emphasise this is a likely adrenal insufficiency/Addison's/Addisonian crisis or emergency AND describe symptoms (vomiting, diarrhoea, dehydration, injury/shock).

Emergency treatment of adrenal crisis

1) **Immediate** 100mg Hydrocortisone i.v. or i.m. injection. **Followed by** 24 hr continuous i.v. infusion of 200mg Hydrocortisone in Glucose 5% **OR** 50mg Hydrocortisone i.v. or i.m. qds (100mg if severely obese).
2) Rapid rehydration with Sodium Chloride 0.9%.
3) Liaise with endocrinology team.

Scan here for further information or search https://www.endocrinology.org/adrenal-crisis

Figure 1.
Example of a European (UK) steroid emergency card (https://www.endocrinology.org/media/3873/steroid-card.pdf).

through patient specific literature and leaflets. Patients should be provided with a supply of IM 100 mg hydrocortisone with counseling provided to patients and carers on its emergency use. In the event of severe illness and/or inability to tolerate oral glucocorticoids; stat IM 100 mg hydrocortisone should be given alongside contact to emergency medical services as these patients may require admission for parenteral hydrocortisone, fluids and stabilization. Further advice and support can be provided by specialist endocrine team and national support organizations such as *The Pituitary Foundation* and *Addison's Self-Help Group* in the UK. Steroids emergency cards (**Figure 1**), bracelets and necklaces are increasingly commonplace in Europe. *The Endocrine Society* suggests that all patients with adrenal insufficiency carry medical alert identification so that medical personnel can be prompted to increase steroids doses to avert adrenal crises and to administer parenteral hydrocortisone immediately in emergency circumstances [4].

An adrenal crisis if a life threating scenario that requires prompt intervention. Data from the *European Adrenal Insufficiency Registry* has shown an incidence rate 7.94 adrenal crises per 100 patient years [19] which is consistent with rates seen in other studies [20]. There are no systematic dose–response studies for the appropriate dosing of hydrocortisone during a crisis therefore management is mostly undertaken on an empirical basis. Underdoing of therapy can be harmful therefore general guidance is to give 100 mg of parenteral hydrocortisone followed by a 200 mg/day infusion or 6 hourly 50 mg boluses alongside appropriate intravenous fluid resuscitation and treatment of the intercurrent illness. To prevent future crises it is important the preceding medical and behavioral factors are explored including medicine concordance and knowledge of sick day rules. It is also recommended that patients with adrenal insufficiency receive an annual influenza vaccine and pneumococcal vaccination above the age of 60, as well as continuing to alert healthcare staff of their steroid dependent status prior to procedures or in light of acute illness [4, 11].

9. Pregnancy and breast feeding

The diagnosis of primary adrenal insufficiency in pregnancy is a rare entity and is a challenge to diagnose due to a degree in overlap in symptomology. The corticotropin stimulation test remains the most appropriate and safe diagnostic tool. A higher minimum post stimulation cortisol is expected during pregnancy and from a small cohort study of healthy pregnant woman levels of 700 nmol/L, 800 nmol/L and 900 nmol/L have been suggested as diagnostic thresholds for the first, second and third trimesters respectively [4]. Timely diagnosis and management of this condition are imperative for reducing maternal/foetal morbidity and mortality.

There is a gradual increase of free cortisol levels during pregnancy with a significant influence of CRH secretion from the placenta peaking in the third trimester (up to 2–3 fold). There is also a notable increase in estrogen driven cortisol binding globulin levels. Therefore an increase in glucocorticoid dosing is expected during pregnancy; with a 20–40% dose increase often necessitated after the 24th week of gestation reflecting the physiological increased cortisol demand in pregnancy [21].

During pregnancy hydrocortisone is the preferable glucocorticoid replacement agent and dexamethasone is best avoided due to its lack of inactivation by 11β-hydroxysteroid dehydrogenase type 2 when traversing the placenta. Reviewing hormone replacement challenging but is best placed by assessing for signs/symptoms of over or under replacement including weight gain/distribution, fatigue, blood pressure and glycaemic control; with recommendation of at least one endocrine clinical review per trimester from *The Endocrine Society* [4]. Patient education and glucocorticoid self-adjustment in relation to sick days rules remain important in the gestational period and advice should be readily available from endocrine specialist teams.

Plasma renin activity is not a reliable measure in judging suitability of Fludrocortisone dosing due to physiological increments in plasma levels during pregnancy. Therefore assessment should include review for signs/symptoms of over or under replacement including weight gain, salt craving, blood pressure and excessive fluid retention. Progesterone has anti-mineralocorticoid effects therefore fludrocortisone doses often need to be increased in the third trimester [11]. However as hydrocortisone exhibits mineralocorticoid activity, an increased dose of hydrocortisone in the second/third trimesters may negate the need to increase the fludrocortisone dose [21].

A delivery care plan should be made in advance from the endocrinologists for the obstetricians. This should involve the administration of a 100 mg parenteral hydrocortisone bolus prior to the active stage of labour followed by 6 hourly 50 mg boluses or a continuous infusion. Cortisol requirements rapidly reduce post-delivery. Patients can be given doubled dosing of gestational hydrocortisone doses in the initial 24-48 hours post-delivery; with prompt down titration back to pre-pregnancy doses if clinically stable [11, 21].

Studies exploring medicines excretion into breastmilk and subsequent effects on infants are rare. Glucocorticoids are expressed in breast milk in minimal amounts and are unlikely to pose any significant harm to breast feeding infants. Therefore in most cases the benefits of replacement therapy will outweigh any potential risk. Greater caution should be employed in those taking high dose steroid therapy i.e. >160 mg daily hydrocortisone or > 40 mg daily prednisolone. In such cases infants should be monitored more closely for potential signs of adrenal suppression and consideration of delaying breast feeding until a few hours post dose administration to minimize exposure.

10. Dosing in special circumstances

There has been minimal clinical research into the effect of exercise or prolonged traveling on patients with adrenal insufficiency. A small randomized-control cross over trial with pre-exercise hydrocortisone revealed no discernable benefits (in metabolic, hormonal or QoL parameters) in short strenuous exercise compared to placebo [22]. Generally dose increments of hydrocortisone or fludrocortisone is not required in exercise regimens and patients should keep to the principles of warming-up, staying well hydrated and warming-down. However with very intense or prolonged exercise (e.g. marathons) or challenging environmental conditions (e.g. hot weather) increased doses may be warranted at 1.5 to 2 times usual dosing during duration of exercise [23, 24]. Patients are encouraged to take extra hydrocortisone with them (or their alternative glucocorticoid medications) when traveling abroad. On long haul flights greater than 12 hours a doubled dose of hydrocortisone is recommended on the day of the flight. Patients should also carry a letter from their endocrinologist with them to enable them to bring their emergency kit along with them. Severe psychological shock such as bereavement or a road traffic accident may also warrant short term doubling of hydrocortisone dosing.

Studies have confirmed changes in the diurnal cortisol pattern in shift workers [25]. Therefore with night shift workers medications should be taken in line with their current sleep–wake cycle with the first dose taken upon waking irrespective if this is in the evening time.

11. Drug interactions

Drugs such as carbamazepine, phenytoin, topiramate and rifampicin induce the hepatic CYP3A4 enzyme which increases cortisol metabolism; grapefruit juice also has a similar effect. Drugs such as ketoconazole, etomidate, abiraterone acetate and tyrosine kinase inhibitors are known to reduce steroidogenesis and lower cortisol levels. Liquorice ingestion can inhibit the 11β-hydroxysteroid dehydrogenase type 2 enzyme leading to cortisol led over-activation of renal mineralocorticoid receptors causing fluid retention, hypertension, hypokalaemia and metabolic alkalosis [11].

On the contrary antiretroviral drugs such as ritonavir are potent enzyme inhibitors and can commonly cause cushingoid features and adrenal suppression. Patients on any interfering medications may need titration of hormone replacement therapy and closer monitoring under endocrinologist review. Additionally it is important to note that those with combined adrenal insufficiency and hypothyroidism should receive glucocorticoid replacement therapy first as proceeding with thyroxine initially can increase cortisol metabolism and precipitate an adrenal crisis.

12. Future perspectives

Although hydrocortisone generally remains the cornerstone of adrenal insufficiency hormone replacement. There have been advancements in delivery modalities including modified released preparations (Plenadren®, Chronocort®) and continuous subcutaneous hydrocortisone infusions (CSHI) for which further comparative RCTs would be beneficial to further explore any benefits in metabolic and QoL parameters. Subcutaneous 100 mg hydrocortisone has also been shown to have similar pharmacokinetics and increased satisfaction rates in comparison to intramuscular delivery in a randomized crossover study [26] and therefore could be considered for increased adoption in emergencies circumstances.

Previously it was common place to manage Cushing's disease with bilateral adrenalectomy with occasional deployment of adrenocortical tissue autotransplantation. This has shown variability in long term graft survival and degree of cortisol production [27, 28]. This is now no longer common practice with advancements in techniques in localizing and resecting autonomous corticotroph pituitary lesions. Successful allotransplantation has also been described to the level of individual case reports including simultaneous kidney-adrenal and kidney-adrenal-pancreas transplantation [29, 30] and a young girl with a successfully functioning intramuscular adrenal allograft at 3 years follow up [31]. Xenotransplantation has been explored in more recent research with good results in pre-clinical studies with transplanted adrenocortical cells displaying the ability to survive, become vascularized and to supersede the hosts' organ in secreting sufficient cortisol levels [32].

There has been growing interest and understanding in the realms of the extraction and reprogramming of pluripotent stem cells (from human embryonic or somatic origins) towards obtaining adrenocortical resembling cells with steroidogenic properties as observed in several pre-clinical studies. Reprogramming can be achieved through the forced expression of steroidogenic factor 1 (SF1) allowing cells the maintained ability to secrete steroid hormones in response to physiological and pharmacological stimuli once transplanted into murine specimens [3]. Encapsulation devices with biocompatible semi-permeable membranes have shown efficacy in type 1 diabetic undergoing islet cell transplantation in sparing the need for immunosuppression [33] which should pave the way for preventing rejection (without need for immunosuppression) from transplantation of adrenocortical tissue regardless of original source. Further research and collaboration is required to translate these therapies into relevant clinical studies.

There are reports that 15–30% of patients can retain some corticosteroid production even years after diagnosis [11]. Individual studies have reviewed the ability to regenerate adrenal function with B-cell depleting therapy and tetracosactide therapy both in isolation and combined. There is some evidence of partial or full response and is an area which may warrant further research [34–36].

Gene therapy is another area of interest in regards to management of 21-hydroxylase deficiency. With the intravenous injection of an adenoviral-Cyp21a1 vector in murine studies have displayed a return to functioning enzyme production and steroidogenesis but the effects appear to be transient [37–40]. It is yet to be seen whether these pre-clinical findings will translate into sustained and effective treatments in humans but is another area with potential for future considerations.

Acknowledgements

I would like to thank the endocrinology department at King's College Hospital NHS Foundation Trust for all their hard work and ongoing support.

Conflict of interest

The authors declare no conflict of interest.

Author details

Michael C. Onyema
King's College Hospital NHS Foundation Trust, London, UK

*Address all correspondence to: michael.onyema@nhs.net

IntechOpen

© 2021 The Author(s). Licensee IntechOpen. This chapter is distributed under the terms of the Creative Commons Attribution License (http://creativecommons.org/licenses/by/3.0), which permits unrestricted use, distribution, and reproduction in any medium, provided the original work is properly cited.

References

[1] Thomas-Addison [Internet]. 2018. Available from: https://www.encyclopedia.com/people/medicine/medicine-biographies/thomas-addison [Accessed: 2021-05-01]

[2] Wass J, et al. Oxford Handbook of Endocrinology and Diabetes. 2nd ed. Oxford University Press; 2014

[3] Liew S, Akker Sam Guasti L, Pittawy JFH. Glucocorticoid replacement therapies: past, present and future. Current Opinion in Endocrine and Metabolic Research. 2019;8:152-159

[4] Bornstein SR, Allolio B, Arlt W, Barthel A, Don-Wauchope A, Hammer GD, Husebye ES, Merke DP, Murad MH, Stratakis CA, Torpy DJ. Diagnosis and Treatment of Primary Adrenal Insufficiency: An Endocrine Society Clinical Practice Guideline. The Journal of Clinical Endocrinology & Metabolism. 2016;101(2):364-389

[5] Javorsky B, Carroll T, Algeciras-Schimnich A, Singh R, Colon-Franco J, Findling J. SAT-390 New Cortisol Threshold for Diagnosis of Adrenal Insufficiency After Cosyntropin Stimulation Testing Using the Elecsys Cortisol II, Access Cortisol, and LC-MS/MS Assays. Journal of the Endocrine Society. 2019;3(1): SAT-390

[6] Deutschbein T, Unger N, Mann K, Petersenn S. Diagnosis of secondary adrenal insufficiency in patients with hypothalamic–pituitary disease: comparison between serum and salivary cortisol during the high-dose short synacthen test. European Journal of Endocrinology. 2009;160(1):9-16

[7] Wallace I, Cunningham S, Lindsay J. The diagnosis and investigation of adrenal insufficiency in adults. Annals of Clinical Biochemistry. 2009;46(5):351-367

[8] Oster H, Challet E, Ott V, Arvat E, Ronald de Kloet E, Dijk D, Lightman S, Vgontzas A, Van Cauter E. The Functional and Clinical Significance of the 24-Hour Rhythm of Circulating Glucocorticoids. Endocrine Reviews. 2017;38:3-45

[9] Kiko N, Kalhan A. Comparison of Various Glucocorticoid Replacement Regimens Used in Chronic Adrenal Insufficiency: A Systematic Review. Dubai Diabetes Endocrinol J. 2020;26:50-68

[10] Ekman B, Fitts D, Marelli C, Murray RD, Quinkler M, Zelissen PMJ. European Adrenal Insufficiency Registry (EU-AIR): a comparative observational study of glucocorticoid replacement therapy. BMC Endocr Disord. 2014;14

[11] Husebye ES, Pearce SH, Krone NP, Kämpe O. Adrenal Insufficiency. The Lancet. 2021;397:613-629

[12] Williams EL, Choudhury S, Tan T, Meeran K. Prednisolone Replacement Therapy Mimics the Circadian Rhythm More Closely Than Other Glucocorticoids. The Journal of Applied Laboratory Medicine. 2016;1:152-161

[13] Smith DJF, Prabhudev H, Choudhury S, Meeran K. Prednisolone has the same cardiovascular risk profile as hydrocortisone in glucocorticoid replacement. Endocrine Connections. 2017;6(8):766-772

[14] Frey KR, Kienitz T, Schulz J, Ventz M, Zopf K, Quinkler M. Prednisolone is associated with a worse bone mineral density in primary adrenal insufficiency. Endocrine Connections. 2018;7(6):811-818

[15] Quinkler M, Ekman B, Marelli C, Uddin S, Zelissen P, Murray RD & on behalf of the EU-AIR Investigators.

Prednisolone is associated with a worse lipid profile than hydrocortisone in patients with adrenal insufficiency. Endocrine Connections. 2017;6(1):1-8

[16] Choudhury S, Tan T, Lazarus K, Meeran K. The use of prednisolone versus dual-release hydrocortisone in the treatment of hypoadrenalism. Endocrine Connections. 2021;10(2):66-76

[17] Oprea A, Bonnet N, Pollé O, Lysy PA. Novel insights into glucocorticoid replacement therapy for pediatric and adult adrenal insufficiency. Therapeutic advances in endocrinology and metabolism. 2019;10:2042018818821294

[18] Gurnell EM, Hunt PJ, Curran SE, Conway CL, Pullenayegum EM, Huppert FA, Compston JE, Herbert J, Chatterjee VKK. Long-Term DHEA Replacement in Primary Adrenal Insufficiency: A Randomized, Controlled Trial. The Journal of Clinical Endocrinology & Metabolism. 2008;93(2):400-409

[19] Quinkler M, Ekman B, Zhang P, Isidori AM, Murray RD; on behalf of the EU-AIR Investigators. Mortality data from the European Adrenal Insufficiency Registry—Patient characterization and associations. Clinical Endocrinology (Oxf). 2018;89:30-35

[20] Puar TH, Stikkelbroeck NM, Smans LC, Zelissen PM, Hermus AR. Adrenal Crisis: Still a Deadly Event in the 21st Century. The American Journal of Medicine. 2016;129(3):339.e1-9

[21] Oliveira D, Lages A, Paiva S, Carrilho F. Treatment of Addison's disease during pregnancy. Endocrinology, diabetes & metabolism case reports. 2018;17-0179

[22] Simunkova K, Jovanovic N, Rostrup E, Methlie P, Øksnes M, Nilsen RM, Hennø H, Tilseth M, Godang K, Kovac A, Løvås K, Husebye ES. Effect of a pre-exercise hydrocortisone dose on short-term physical performance in female patients with primary adrenal failure. European Journal of Endocrinology. 2016;174(1):97-105

[23] Dr Rob Andrews. How to stay on top of exercise [Internet]. 2018. Available from: https://www.addisonsdisease.org.uk/how-to-stay-on-top-of-an-exercise-programme-with-addisons-disease [Accessed: 2021-05-30]

[24] Dineen R, Thompson CJ, Sherlock M. Adrenal crisis: prevention and management in adult patients. Therapeutic advances in endocrinology and metabolism. 2019;10, 2042018819848218

[25] Li J, Bidlingmaier M, Petru R, Pedrosa GF, Loerbroks A, Angerer P. Impact of shift work on the diurnal cortisol rhythm: a one-year longitudinal study in junior physicians. Journal of occupational medicine and toxicology. 2018;13,23

[26] Hahner S, Burger-Stritt S, Allolio B. Subcutaneous hydrocortisone administration for emergency use in adrenal insufficiency. European Journal of Endocrinology. 2013;169(2):147-154

[27] Hardy JD, Moore DO, Langford HG. Cushing's disease today. Late follow-up of 17 adrenalectomy patients with emphasis on eight with adrenal autotransplants. Annals of surgery. 1985;201(5):595-603

[28] Hardy JD. Surgical management of Cushing's syndrome with emphasis on adrenal autotransplantation. Annals of surgery. 1978;188(3):290-307

[29] Dubernard JM, Cloix P, Tajra LC, Alduglihan W, Borson F, Lefrançois N, Martin X. Simultaneous adrenal gland and kidney allotransplantation after

synchronous bilateral renal cell carcinoma: a case report. Transplant Proc. 1995;27(1):1320-1321

[30] Vouillarmet J, Buron F, Houzard C, Carlier MC, Chauvet C, Brunet M, Thivolet C, Morelon E, Badet L. The first simultaneous kidney-adrenal gland-pancreas transplantation: outcome at 1 year. American Journal of Transplantation. 2013;13(7):1905-1909

[31] Grodstein E, Hardy MA, Goldstein MJ. A case of human intramuscular adrenal gland transplantation as a cure for chronic adrenal insufficiency. American Journal of Transplantation. 2010;10(2):431-433

[32] Ruiz-Babot G, Hadjidemetriou I, King PJ, Guasti L. New directions for the treatment of adrenal insufficiency. Frontiers in endocrinology. 2015;6,70

[33] Ludwig B, Reichel A, Steffen A, Zimerman B, Schally AV, Block NL, Colton CK, Ludwig S, Kersting S, Bonifacio E, Solimena M, Gendler Z, Rotem A, Barkai U, Bornstein SR. Transplantation of human islets without immunosuppression. Proc Natl Acad Sci USA. 2013;110(47):19054-19058

[34] Simon SHS, Mitchell AL, Bennett S, King P, Chandran S, Nag S, Chen S, Smith BR, Isaacs JD, Vaidya B: Adrenal Steroidogenesis after B Lymphocyte Depletion Therapy in New-Onset Addison's Disease. The Journal of Clinical Endocrinology & Metabolism. 2012;97(10):E1927–E1932

[35] Napier C, Gan EH, Mitchell AL, Gilligan LC, Rees DA, Moran C, Chatterjee K, Vaidya B, James RA, Mamoojee Y, Ashwell S, Arlt W, Pearce SHS. Residual Adrenal Function in Autoimmune Addison's Disease— Effect of Dual Therapy With Rituximab and Depot Tetracosactide. The Journal of Clinical Endocrinology & Metabolism. 2020;105(4): e1250–e1259

[36] Gan EH, MacArthur K, Mitchell AL, Hughes BA, Perros P, Ball SG, James RA, Quinton R, Chen S, Furmaniak J, Arlt W, Pearce SH. Residual adrenal function in autoimmune Addison's disease: improvement after tetracosactide (ACTH1-24) treatment. The Journal of Clinical Endocrinology & Metabolism. 2014;99(1):111-118

[37] Tajima T, Okada T, Ma XM, Ramsey W, Bornstein S, Aguilera G. Restoration of adrenal steroidogenesis by adenovirus-mediated transfer of human cytochromeP450 21-hydroxylase into the adrenal gland of 21-hydroxylase-deficient mice. Gene Therapy. 1999 Nov;6(11):1898-1903

[38] Perdomini M, Dos Santos C, Goumeaux C, Blouin V, Bougnères P. An AAVrh10-CAG-CYP21-HA vector allows persistent correction of 21-hydroxylase deficiency in a Cyp21-/- mouse model. Gene Therapy. 2017;24(5):275-281

[39] Markmann S, De BP, Reid J, Jose CL, Rosenberg JB, Leopold PL, Kaminsky SM, Sondhi D, Pagovich O, Crystal RG. Biology of the Adrenal Gland Cortex Obviates Effective Use of Adeno-Associated Virus Vectors to Treat Hereditary Adrenal Disorders. Human Gene Therapy. 2018;29(4):403-412

[40] Naiki Y, Miyado M, Horikawa R, Katsumata N, Onodera M, Pang S, Ogata T, Fukami M. Extra-adrenal induction of Cyp21a1 ameliorates systemic steroid metabolism in a mouse model of congenital adrenal hyperplasia. Endocrine Journal. 2016;63(10):897-904

Milton Keynes UK
Ingram Content Group UK Ltd.
UKHW051858070923
428268UK00010B/191